"Dr. Kirschenbaum's book is packed with scientifically sound, balanced, practical, and reader-friendly information and guidance—a truly winning combination. His no-nonsense approach is invaluable for anyone who is serious about losing weight and maintaining the loss for a lifetime. Congratulations, Dr. Kirschenbaum, for having the courage to tell it as it is! His concept of a 'healthy obsession' includes persistence, vigilance, consistency, passion, and focus—key factors for lifetime success."

—Judy E. Marshel, Ph.D., R.D., C.D.N.
Former Senior Nutritionist at Weight Watchers International
Nutrition Therapist for the Live Light—Live Right *Weight Control Program*
at Brookdale University Hospital & Medical Center

"As Dr. Kirschenbaum continues to be a wise guiding light in helping all scientists understand the complex medical, behavioral, and emotional challenges of obesity treatment, his books for the public are profound, pragmatic, and personable. I can find no better compendium of facts and clear practical advice for overweight people than this one. The value to all who read *The Wellspring Weight Loss Plan* will be self-evident from the very first chapter and I have no doubt that the *Wellspring Plan* will be used as a reference book in obesity treatment for decades to come. No wonder countless obesity experts entrust their patients to Dr. Kirschenbaum."

—John Rabkin, M.D.
Co-Director, Pacific Laparoscopy (San Francisco, CA)
Former Associate Professor of Surgery,
Oregon Health and Sciences University
Fellow, American College of Surgery
Researcher/Author, Numerous Scientific Publications About Surgery
for the Treatment of Obesity

"A terrific book filled with practical steps   it
those crazy diets; follow these 8 steps a   :-
cess."

D1502159

—John Fore)
Professor of Medicine and Director, Beh
Baylor College of Medicine, Houston, TX

"As a dietitian and weight loss counselor for twenty-seven years, I have seen that individuals require individual approaches for successful weight loss, while consuming healthy low-fat, high-fiber, high-quality foods (including carbs!), and moving more daily. The success stories in this book prove that Dr. Kirschenbaum has a formula for weight loss that really works! The comprehensive cognitive-behavioral approach he uses, incorporating healthy eating and exercise, has helped countless individuals to lose weight and turn their lives around."

—Georgia Kostas, M.P.H., R.D., L.D.
Nutrition Consultant
Author, The Cooper Clinic Solution to the Diet Revolution

"At last, a scientifically grounded, practical guide to safe and long-term weight loss—one that might help put a stop to the insanity surrounding low-carb fad diets. Dr. Kirschenbaum has been a distinguished researcher and consultant for thirty years in the field of weight management, and he has helped thousands of people lose weight safely."

—Rob Smith, Ph.D.
Psychologist, Waltham, MA

"Dr. Kirschenbaum understands precisely the challenges that dieters face—and how to help them. He not only explains how to eat and exercise, but he tackles the question that other books never touch: 'How do we motivate ourselves to do what we need to do?' With his research-based techniques and touching case examples, readers can find the inspiration and skills they need to succeed at losing weight and keeping it off."

—Eileen Rosendahl, Ph.D.
Coordinator of Outreach and Education, Center for Weight Management,
North Shore-Long Island Jewish Health System
Assistant Professor of Psychiatry and Behavioral Sciences,
Albert Einstein College of Medicine

"In a world filled with bogus, fad diets it is nice to see an experienced psychologist using his research and clinical background to offer the general public sound advice."

—Jennifer Bremer, M.D.
Medical Director, Eating Disorders Program,
Department of Child and Adolescent Psychiatry,
Psychopharmacology Clinic, University of Chicago

"Professor Kirschenbaum's approach has helped a great many of my patients lose weight and keep it off for years. This book is the latest word on how to lose weight from a master therapist and scientist."

—Frances J. Langdon, M.D.
Clinical Instructor, Board Certified in Internal Medicine,
Northwestern University Medical School

THE WELLSPRING WEIGHT LOSS PLAN

The Simple, Scientific, & Sustainable Approach of the World's Most Successful Weight Loss Programs for Overweight Young People—and How You Can Achieve Lifelong Success with It

With more than fifty amazingly delicious and easy recipes from the chefs of Wellspring, the developers of remarkably effective weight loss programs for overweight teenagers (Wellspring Academies and Wellspring Camps) and adults (Wellspring Retreats).

THE WELLSPRING WEIGHT LOSS PLAN

The Simple, Scientific, & Sustainable Approach of the World's Most Successful Weight Loss Programs for Overweight Young People—and How You Can Achieve Lifelong Success with It

DANIEL S. KIRSCHENBAUM, PH.D.

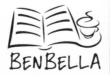

BenBella

BENBELLA BOOKS, INC.
Dallas, Texas

Nothing written in this book should be viewed as a substitute for competent medical care. Also, you should not undertake any changes in diet or exercise patterns without first consulting your physician if you are currently being treated for any risk factor related to heart disease, high blood pressure or adult onset diabetes, or if you have food allergies.

The Wellspring Weight Loss Plan was originally titled *The Healthy Obsession Program*. This special edition is a paperback version exclusively printed for the Wellspring Academies.

BenBella Books, Inc.
10300 N. Central Expressway, Suite 400
Dallas, TX 75231
www.benbellabooks.com
Send feedback to feedback@benbellabooks.com

Printed in the United States of America
10 9 8 7 6 5 4 3 2 1

Proofreading by Jessica Keet, Stacia Seaman, and Andrew Lucas
Cover design by Faceout Studio
Text design and composition by John Reinhardt Book Design
Printed by Bang Printing

Library of Congress Cataloging-in-Publication Data is available for this title.
ISBN 978-1-935618-77-5

Distributed by Perseus Distribution
www.perseusdistribution.com

To place orders through Perseus Distribution:
Tel: (800) 343-4499
Fax: (800) 351-5073
E-mail: orderentry@perseusbooks.com

Significant discounts for bulk sales are available.
Please contact Glenn Yeffeth at glenn@benbellabooks.com or (214) 750-3628.

DEDICATION

To the thousands of people who have embraced the Wellspring Plan, *and especially to the parents who have trusted the author and other members of the staff of Wellspring's programs to help their overweight children, overweight teens, and themselves make radical changes in their lives; we honor that trust and aspire to earn it every day.*

Contents

1 The Wellspring Plan: 8 Steps to Success 1

2 Step 1: Make the Decision 27

3 Step 2: Know the Enemy—Your Biology 61

4 Step 3: Eat to Lose 77

5 Step 4: Find Lovable Foods that Love You Back 123

6 Step 5: Move to Lose 137

7 Step 6: Self-Monitor and Plan Consistently 173

8 Step 7: Understand and Manage Stress—With and Without Food 201

9 Step 8: Use Slump Busters to Overcome Slumps 227

10 The Wellspring Plan for Overweight Children and Teens: A Parents' Guide to Healthier, Happier Children 245

11 Recipes from Wellspring Chefs 259

References 301

About the Author 310

The Wellspring Plan:
8 Steps to Success

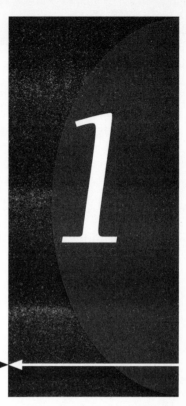

THIS BOOK WILL DO TWO THINGS for you. First, you will learn about *Wellspring's 3-1-8 Plan* and how it can help you live a healthier and better life. Second, you will increase your motivation to succeed because of the surprising simplicity of the approach, the compelling nature of the evidence that supports it, and the convincing stories of those who have used it to make dramatic changes in their lives.

This chapter will introduce you to the *3-1-8 Wellspring Plan*. This approach has led thousands of your fellow weight controllers, including me, to safe and permanent weight loss. You will find that the *Wellspring Plan* encourages you to find foods you love that love you back (without feeling hungry) and ways of increasing your everyday movement (without training for a marathon)—plus, you'll do this with more comfort, satisfaction, and success than you ever could have imagined. The *Wellspring Plan* isn't a specific diet; it is a pathway to a better life. You'll find plenty of bumps along this road; but, through the *Wellspring Plan*, you'll learn how to overcome the inevitable obstacles and master one of life's most difficult challenges.

Basics of the 3-1-8 Wellspring Plan

You've seen them.

You've talked to them.

You've probably even touched them.

Successful weight controllers are out there. They have disappointments, failings, and joys, just like you. Research shows that most of them have lost weight and put it right back on many times before succeeding permanently. They've crossed over to the other side, but they've also discovered that weight loss doesn't cure all ills, nor does it open every door to success and love. If you ask any of them, though, they will tell you that as difficult as it is to lose weight and keep it off, it's much more difficult to live the life of an overweight person.

This book will demonstrate how they did it and how you can do it, as well. I am actually one of those who have crossed to the other side. I lost thirty pounds and have kept it off for forty years. In this book, I will help you learn how you can do the same thing. This approach was developed by my colleagues and me after years of research and leans heavily on the scientific efforts of hundreds of other researchers who have studied how to help people lose weight and keep it off permanently.

The *3-1-8* approach helped create the world's largest and most successful programs for overweight young people, *Wellspring* (wellspringweightloss.com). In 2004, Ryan Craig, the founding president of *Wellspring*, had obtained substantial funding from what is now the largest behavioral healthcare organization in the United States, CRC Health Group. This funding allowed Ryan to hire me and obtain the consultation of other experienced scientists from many major research universities. We created the *3-1-8 Wellspring Plan* and our programs grew in five years from two camps to twelve *Wellspring Camps,* two *Wellspring Academies* (the world's first boarding schools for overweight young people), four community programs (*Wellspring Fit Clubs*), and *Wellspring Retreats* (eight-day spa-vacation-workshops for overweight adults). In the summer of 2010, Wellspring programs helped more than 1,000 young people (and their families) learn how to use the Wellspring Plan to become successful weight controllers.

I've used the same approach in my clinic in Chicago (Center for Behavioral Medicine, ChicagoCBM.com) help people of all ages master the challenges of weight loss for more than twenty-five years.

We're asked by media reporters and potential clients all the time, "What makes your approach special? Why does it work so well?" Or, to put it in a gustatory perspective, "What's your 'special sauce'?" The sauce is the *3-1-8* plan (three simple behavioral goals; one overarching mission; and eight steps to get there):

3 Simple Behavioral Goals

1. Eat very little fat. (aim for zero fat grams per day, accept 20g per day)
2. Stay quite active, accumulating at least 10,000 steps per day on a pedometer (or the equivalent in energy expenditure).
3. Self-monitor (write down in a journal) 100% of your eating and steps (and exercise).

1 Overarching Goal

To develop a healthy obsession.

Weight controllers face enormous challenges from our obesogenic culture and from their own biological barriers to success. To overcome these challenges, research shows that a very consistent pattern of behavior and focusing seems necessary: a healthy obsession. When you read the following definition, you'll see that all athletes strive for this critical pattern of thinking and behaving, as well. Sometimes psychologists call healthy obsessions "positive addictions" or "adaptive perfectionism." *The Wellspring Weight Loss Plan* will help you do this as comfortably and happily as possible.

A *healthy obsession* **is a sustained preoccupation with the planning and execution of target behaviors to reach a healthy goal.**

8 Steps to Develop and Maintain Your Healthy Obsession

1. Make the Decision
2. Know the Enemy—Your Biology
3. Eat to Lose
4. Find Lovable Foods that Love You Back
5. Move to Lose
6. Self-Monitor and Plan Consistently
7. Understand and Manage Stress—With and Without Food
8. Use Slump Busters to Overcome Slumps

You will understand, after reviewing the following material, why the development of a healthy obsession about weight loss is the overarching goal of the *Wellspring Plan*—and why developing a healthy obsession is so critical for you. The remainder of this chapter will introduce you to each of the eight steps found essential by many masterful weight controllers in developing their healthy obsessions. The following eight chapters expand these ideas and present case examples of how people have benefited from taking each of the eight steps. The penultimate chapter will describe how to use this approach with children, essentially a mini parent's guide to using the *Wellspring Plan* with overweight young people. The final chapter presents more than fifty fabulous recipes for creating very low-fat, healthful taste sensations.

Healthy Obsession

In a recent guidebook for parents of overweight young people that I cowrote with two of my Wellspring colleagues, we defined a *healthy obsession* as I mentioned above as "a sustained preoccupation with the planning and execution of target behaviors to reach a healthy goal." The word "obsession" refers to the persistence of these thoughts, their sustained quality despite distractions from life, and their impact on action. Healthy obsessions compel actions to achieve healthy goals. When you have a good, solid healthy obsession, you will feel driven to get a good level of activity every day and to eat according to your program, every time you eat and every day. A healthy obsession can also help you overcome various forms of resistance to permanent weight loss. As will be described in detail in Chapter 3, your body contains billions of hungry fat cells that naturally resist weight loss. The resistance of these cells is just one of the many biological forces that do not want you to lose weight and keep it off. Unfortunately, these forces never go on vacation, nor do they give partial credit for moderate, albeit sincere, effort.

To subdue these primal biological forces, you must take extreme measures. Not only does your biology resist permanent weight loss, but your lifestyle probably resists it, as well. You've developed habits that are comfortable for you. Some of these habits, including the way you order food at restaurants and the way you move on a daily basis, can interfere with successful weight loss. You must develop compelling ways of thinking about weight control—including a tremendous focus on consistency of eating, movement, and exercise—to overcome these barriers to success.

I developed this concept of a healthy obsession for weight controllers based on several decades spent directing weight loss programs and conducting research studies on this topic. I have done this work at the University of Rochester in New York, the University of Wisconsin in Madison, Northwestern University Medical School in Chicago, the Center for Behavioral Medicine & Sport Psychology in Chicago, La Rabida Children's Hospital in Chicago, Swedish Covenant Hospital in Chicago, and for *Wellspring*. Thousands of participants in these programs have become masterful weight controllers because they developed healthy obsessions about weight loss. The research evidence about this is extremely convincing. Before I present a version of that science, it would be useful for you to know how some of my clients developed and maintained their healthy obsessions.

Case Examples of Healthy Obsessions in Action

Table 1.1 describes my current clients who have attempted to change their lives for at least three months. A review of the table shows that twenty out of twenty-one of them have made significant progress toward successful weight control. They have achieved an average weight loss of forty-seven pounds, with 82% of them reaching their weight loss goals (within 20% of an ideal weight). The scientific literature rarely includes weight losses of this magnitude. As you read the descriptions of four of these clients and their healthy obsessions, consider how their approach to the problem differs from the one you currently use.

Sam[1]: Stringent, Committed, and Determined. Sam was plagued by more than fifty excess pounds for more than forty years. This excess weight made him feel lousy about himself and took its toll physically. Now seventy-four, Sam has undergone both back surgery and a hip replacement, and suffered from other maladies his doctors attribute to the weight problem and a lack of conditioning. More than five years ago he began working in one of my clinics and was extremely consistent in his self-monitoring: he wrote down everything he ate and his daily activity patterns. He was willing to take a close look at his life and find ways of changing it.

---

[1] All of the case materials in this book are based directly on people whom I have helped during the past thirty years. The names and other details in each case and those throughout the book have been changed to protect confidentiality.

One of the hallmarks of Sam's healthy obsession, in addition to his remarkably consistent self-monitoring, is his refusal to accept eating problems without closely analyzing the factors that caused them. These analyses always include deciding how he could avoid or limit such problems in the future.

Sam's journey toward successful weight control has not been without its obstacles, but his willingness to deal with the realities of his eating situation has made his healthy obsession permanent. Sam has experienced difficulty over the years during emotionally trying times, sometimes resulting in late-night binge-eating. But over time he has learned to minimize the potential damage of his binges by eating only low-fat foods, such as low-fat popcorn and bagels. He has also learned to handle his tendency to binge in the middle of the night by allowing himself only to drink liquids at that time. He has remained true to this commitment, with a few exceptions, always stopping to examine and understand those times he has faltered. Sam is committed to permanent weight loss and will not allow himself to ignore the impact of his own behaviors. He will maintain his self-monitoring, keep moving, and keep trying to solve the problems that interfere with his life. Although Sam's weight is ten pounds higher today than he would like it to be, it is still forty-five pounds lower than it was five years ago.

Al: Success with Soup. Al's younger brother recently died of complications related to super-morbid obesity. This tragedy, as well as Al's substantially failing health, led him to undertake a major effort to reduce his 410 pounds to a weight closer to his 175-pound ideal. Al has developed a remarkable healthy obsession that has allowed him to focus consistently on the details of his eating (via self-monitoring and regular meetings with me)—and has produced a weight loss of 180 pounds!

Al set a variety of goals during the course of the past year that have helped him keep focused. He wears a pedometer and attempts to achieve ten thousand steps per day on that pedometer. He bought a treadmill and tries to spend at least a half-hour a day on the machine. He records the amount of fat he consumes every day and attempts to limit it to less than fifteen fat grams. He also records calories and tries to consume fewer than two thousand per day. At the end of every week and every month he calculates the percentage of times that he achieved his goals. We discuss these percentages and make plans to help him improve them.

					WITHIN 20%
CLIENT	CURRENT AGE	OCCUPATION	DURATION OF TREATMENT	WEIGHT CHANGE	OF GOAL WEIGHT?

TABLE 1.1
DR. KIRSCHENBAUM'S CURRENT CLIENTS' WEIGHT CHANGES

CLIENT	CURRENT AGE	OCCUPATION	DURATION OF TREATMENT	WEIGHT CHANGE	WITHIN 20% OF GOAL WEIGHT?
A	74	pharmacist	5 yrs.	-45	yes
B	45	artist	1.5 yrs.	-40	no
C	56	lawyer	1 yr.	-172	yes
D	45	manager, business	1 yr.	-35	yes
E	53	executive, business	1 yr.	-50	no
F	44	manager, business	2.2 yrs.	-67	yes
G	33	banker	4 mos.	-40	yes
H	70	secretary, retired	2 yrs.	-32	yes
I	29	clerk, student	6 mos.	-28	n/a
J	38	homemaker	3 mos.	-10	n/a
K	37	real estate broker	10 mos.	-43	yes
L	40	computer sales manager	6 mos.	-57	n/a
M	50	librarian	1.8 yrs.	-27	yes
N	55	executive, business	2.2 yrs.	-125	yes
O	33	lawyer	2 yrs.	-50	yes
P	32	driver, delivery	4 mos.	-30	yes
Q	40	priest	5 yrs.	-20	no
R	53	architect	4 yrs.	-30	yes
S	59	physician	6 mos.	-60	n/a
T	44	nurse	6 mos.	-25	yes
U	49	lawyer	1.1 yrs.	-40	yes

* n/a =not applicable; achievement of goal weight was not expected for these clients (morbidly obese) in less than 1 year.

SUMMARY: Average weight loss = 47 lbs; 82% of clients achieved weight loss goals (within 20% of ideal; excluding morbidly obese clients who had not participated for one year).

One distinguishing aspect of Al's healthy obsession concerns a soup/ stew concoction that perhaps only he would really enjoy. Al's soups include everything except the kitchen sink. He starts with cans of soup and adds items such as fat-free hot dogs and a variety of spices. He also typically includes cans of vegetables to thicken the soup, including his personal favorite, baby lima beans. He finds that eating fairly large quantities of the soup helps fill him up and keep him focused on what he is trying to do. He feels safe when eating his soup and becomes concerned when he goes to restaurants or to other people's houses for dinner. Al's concern and focus typify a healthy obsession with weight loss. You need to be both consistently focused and consistently anxious if you face high-risk situations or deviate from your plans.

Mary: A Healthy Kind of Pressure. Mary has a good eye for detail, as do most good librarians. She has used her detail-oriented style to develop a very effective healthy obsession on weight control. She self-monitors carefully and easily, noting when she tends to eat higher-fat foods and when she fails to work out according to her goals. She has made very consistent changes in both her breakfasts and her lunches, finding it easier to control the fat content and the quantity of lunch when she brings her own.

Mary has also attempted to get herself to the gym, particularly on days when she doesn't work. In her job as a librarian she has made it a habit of walking library patrons to the location of the item they need or to the computer, where they can do their own research.

She has maintained her healthy obsession by realizing that problems in eating can be viewed as problems to be solved rather than instances of cheating or minor tragedies. She continues self-monitoring even at the times when she is struggling with the rate of her weight loss. Mary shares a feature of healthy obsessions with many other successful weight controllers: unhappiness and discomfort if she doesn't stick to her low-fat diet on a particular day, or if she fails to achieve her exercise goals for a certain week. Mary has found that she must put that kind of pressure on herself by keeping these goals important enough to demand her attention every day, feeling good about achieving them, but anxious and concerned when she fails to reach them.

Ann: A Commitment to Exercise. Ann has four children and a part-time job as a nurse, but her busy life included room for focusing very carefully on weight loss over a period of six months. Ann set the goal of no more than twelve fat grams per day because she knew that her biology was particularly resistant to effective weight loss. This stringent goal forced her to focus very carefully on food selection both at home and when eating out. She was also determined to get on her treadmill every single day, no matter what was going on with the kids or work or anything else.

Over those six months she fulfilled these goals remarkably well. On the few occasions she failed to use her treadmill for at least a half-hour, she felt anxious, concerned, and unhappy about the situation. In other words, Ann's healthy obsession meant she didn't make excuses for failing to achieve her goals, but redoubled her efforts to decrease the chance of that happening again. Ann is very happy having lost twenty-five pounds and having gotten close to her goal weight, but she knows staying focused, amazingly consistent, and committed are at the heart of the healthy obsession that has allowed her to succeed.

These four individuals illustrate several aspects of healthy obsessions, but all maintain a clear and powerful commitment. A healthy obsession is much more than simple concern or worry about something; it is a dramatic emphasis on that aspect of one's life, so that if it is denied in some way on a particular day the individual feels uncomfortable enough to take action to fix the problem. In addition, those who develop active healthy obsessions about their weight demand consistency from themselves in how they eat, how they move, and the degree to which they pay attention to the details of their eating and movement. These are not people who regularly make exceptions. They may occasionally experience lapses, but they take steps to solve their problems immediately, energized by their strong commitments and sense of urgency about staying true to their commitments.

You'll find many specifics about how to eat, exercise, and manage stress using a healthy obsession in this book. To get a feel for what this looks like, let's consider some key aspects of what a healthy obsession is and is not.

A healthy obsession *IS*:

- Knowing that your biology has turned against you and does not go on vacations or cut you slack because "you've had a rough day"
- Accepting the tough goal of eating as little fat as possible every day
- Knowing that "the devil is in the details" so that writing down all food eaten is critical

- Understanding that everything counts—*everything*
- Being unwilling to accept permission, even from yourself, to over-indulge
- Making plans to help yourself stick with the program at parties, restaurants, and on trips
- Analyzing lapses in order to prevent the same problem from happening tomorrow
- Refusing to allow lapses to become relapses
- Refusing to let a number on a scale prevent you from persisting
- Feeling anxious if goals (for eating, exercising, journaling, etc.) are not met
- Accepting the idea that exercise every day is the only way and doing it, even when you don't feel like it
- Being an active problem solver, oriented to take action, not just to analyze

A healthy obsession *IS NOT*:

- Seeking moderation in all things
- Giving yourself permission to deviate from the program because of moods, stress, holidays, or vacations
- Waltzing into a high-risk situation (like a party or a Mexican restaurant) without a plan
- Making lame excuses for major lapses
- Allowing lapses to turn into relapses
- Feeling just fine when goals are sometimes not met
- Getting thrown into a major tailspin because a number on a scale is too high
- Wallowing in self-pity
- Getting discouraged and overwhelmed

Research Supporting the Importance of Healthy Obsessions for Weight Loss

Many scientific studies have shown that healthy obsessions help people lose weight. For example, researchers have identified a group of four thousand people who lost an average of sixty pounds and kept it off for an average of six years (these four thousand people constitute the National Weight Control Registry). What they learned is that these masters of weight control did not succeed on their first attempts. In fact, they had each lost and regained an average of 270 pounds. A related survey found that most masters of weight control had tried to lose weight permanently at least five times before taking it off and keeping it off. When asked to compare their successes with their failures, they stressed that they used more *extreme approaches* in their successful attempts. More than 60% incorporated a much stricter diet (with much less fat), while more than 80% exercised far more. In fact, these masters reported exercising the equivalent of walking four miles a day. This places them in the top 5% of Americans for the amount and frequency of exercising.

Perhaps the most consistent finding over the past thirty years in weight loss literature is that when people attend professionally conducted weight loss therapy, they usually persist and succeed at losing weight almost every week. Two studies randomly assigned people to groups in which they received either long-term or short-term professional behavioral weight loss therapy. In both studies, the groups that received a longer course of treatment—for example forty weeks versus twenty weeks—lost far more weight. Attending weekly sessions helps people focus on the details of their eating, greatly increases their tendency to self-monitor consistently, and in other ways promotes the development of healthy obsessions.

In a series of studies, psychologist Dr. Michael Perri and his colleagues from the University of Florida found that almost any effort that consistently focused the attention of their clients on the process of losing weight improved the maintenance of weight loss. Comparing different types of booster sessions held weekly over six months, they found that sessions focused on relapse prevention or problem solving did not help maintain weight losses any better than did those focused on discussion of general weight loss issues. They also learned that any kind of contact with their clients—such as sending postcards or making brief phone calls, regardless of the content—improved their clients' abilities to maintain weight loss as compared to people who did not receive such attention.

My colleagues and I conducted two studies during the holiday season (Thanksgiving through New Year in 1997) that yielded similar results. For example, we found that people who received daily mailings about weight loss and an additional phone call from their therapist once a week lost weight even during the challenging holiday season.

Another group of people who did not receive mailings or the phone call, but who continued to attend sessions, gained an average of one pound a week during the holidays. The successful people maintained their consistency of self-monitoring at a very high level, whereas the others, without the extra attention, decreased their consistency to a substantially lower level. Another research team found that when weight controllers were allowed to self-monitor (record everything they ate), they lost twice as much weight and maintained those losses far better than those who were not allowed to self-monitor.

Many other reputable studies support the value of a healthy obsession for successful weight loss. For example, people who have greater stability in their lives because of their jobs, financial situations, and mental health succeed more often than those with unstable personal and work situations. Some studies even find that older adults—those over sixty—tend to succeed more often than their middle-aged counterparts in professional weight loss programs. One good explanation for these findings is that greater stability in life allows weight controllers to focus more clearly on developing very consistent patterns—a key element in healthy obsessions.

The Wellspring Weight Loss Plan Versus Moderation

You have undoubtedly read other scientifically oriented diet books that encourage you to eat well and stay active. The problem is that this advice has not gone far enough. Moderation just won't do. I can't stress enough that it takes an extreme approach to tame the biological and behavioral forces that have prevented you from succeeding in past efforts at losing weight. It takes consistency, persistence, and constant attention to details to achieve success. Moreover, it is important to be unhappy when goals are not achieved, as such unhappiness serves as a powerful motivating force.

The research just reviewed clearly shows the critical role of healthy obsessions for success in weight loss. When you develop your healthy obsession you will feel well-focused and driven toward consistency every day. A moderation approach would allow your fat cells the wiggle room they need to gobble up fat more easily and regain lost weight. Almost every day new studies appear that support this position. For example, in a recent issue of the journal *Health Psychology*, Dr. Perri and his colleagues (the University of Florida researchers mentioned above) reported a study that included 379 sedentary adults who wanted to become more active and fit. Half of the participants were asked to walk for thirty minutes three to four days per week, while the other half of the group were asked to walk for the same duration five to seven days per week. Dr. Perri and his colleagues believed that the moderate approach should have worked better than the extreme approach. They expected that the prescription for three to four days per week would lead to more walking over time. The healthy obsession approach, however, suggests that exercising every day should improve focus and lead to more consistent exercising over the long haul. Sure enough, over the six-month period examined in this study, the more extreme prescription led to 53% more walking than the moderate approach.

A study by psychologist Dr. Eric Stice of Stanford University made a related point about dietary behavior. Stice followed a large sample of sixteen- to nineteen-year-olds over nine months. He found that most of these adolescents reported regularly practicing at least one dietary behavior (for example, consciously reducing the amount of food eaten in order to lose weight). However, his most important finding was that "moderate levels of dieting were associated with weight gain and more extreme forms of dieting were associated with weight loss."

Stice's female extreme dieters, for example, regularly used eighteen out of nineteen possible dietary behaviors in order to try to lose weight. Moderate dieters reported using only half of these dietary behaviors.

Of course, you will need more detailed directions in order to develop your own *Wellspring Plan*. By taking each of the eight steps in the *Wellspring Plan* seriously and engaging in them fully, you, too, can reap the many benefits of this approach. To those who wonder if a healthy obsession sounds a bit extreme, think about this:

Extremism in pursuit of permanent lifestyle change is no vice.
Moderation in defense of failure to change is no virtue.

Let's now take a look at short summaries of the eight steps to successful weight loss so that you have an idea of what to expect.

THE 8 STEPS OF THE WELLSPRING PLAN

1. Make the Decision
2. Know the Enemy—Your Biology
3. Eat to Lose:
   - Very Low Fat
   - Controlled Sugar
   - Frequent Protein
   - Low Density
   - High Fiber
   - Eat Your Calories—Don't Drink Them
   - Calorie Consciousness
4. Find Lovable Foods that Love You Back
5. Move to Lose
6. Self-Monitor and Plan Consistently
7. Understand and Manage Stress—With and Without Food
8. Use Slump Busters to Overcome Slumps

The 8 Steps: A Summary

STEP 1: Make the Decision

You have undoubtedly heard the statement "to not decide is to decide." This applies beautifully to weight loss. You probably know from experience that if you decide not to think about weight loss for a while, you will gain weight—not maintain it. The fact that you are reading this book indicates you are interested in something more than maintenance of your current weight; you have either already decided to lose weight or at least are thinking about making a genuine commitment to lose weight permanently.

Where does weight loss rank in your list of priorities at this very moment? Is it lower in importance than your work? Than your family? Than your hobbies? Or is it the single most important thing in your life? Most successful weight controllers list weight loss near the top of their priorities, usually higher than hobbies—sometimes more important than their jobs. They want improved looks, health, self-esteem, and better choices in clothes. What do you want from this effort? How hard are you willing to work for it?

Even if you can maximize your commitment to weight loss, it takes far more than simply the desire to lose weight. You can have a burning, unquenchable desire to be the best basketball player in the universe. But if you decide to pursue this goal by shooting free throws backward, you are doomed before you start. If you want to lose weight but don't know what science has taught us about how to do it effectively, your back is turned toward your goal. Substantial commitment is needed for any of the other seven steps in the *Wellspring Plan* to work. It is the engine for this particular machine.

STEP 2: Know the Enemy—Your Biology

Since humanity took its collective first steps, perhaps some 200,000 years ago, we have managed to use our big brains to overcome our puny bodies. Many animal species are stronger, faster, and more capable of handling dramatic changes in weather. Our brains, however, have allowed us to create a world to suit our bodies. This unprecedented success as a species has meant that evolution has left our bodies alone for hundreds of thousands of years. Why fix something that isn't broken?

So our bodies may still "think" we spend most of our days actively hunting and gathering, eating insects and wild berries and every once in a while consuming a source of high-fat food like deer or rabbit. Does this sound anything like your current life? I doubt it. Forty-four percent of Americans eat out for at least one meal every single week. Obesity has emerged just in the last one hundred years, primarily in the industrialized countries of the world. Your personal weight problem is no indication that the entire species has a weight problem. For hundreds of thousands of years our bodies have encouraged the storage of fat in order to help us survive the rigors of our cave ancestors' lifestyle. In other words, your body wants you to gain weight, not lose it.

BIOLOGY IS NOT DESTINY

Every athlete has to transform his or her body against the body's will. Consider the case of runners. Most marathoners average forty miles or so per week in the period prior to the big run. World-class marathoners average one hundred miles per week. Do you think the elite marathoners really love spending all that time pounding their bodies into shape for their races? It's incredibly hard work and demands enormous commitment, time, money, and effort. These runners might prefer spending more time on a couch drinking beer and munching potato chips. But committed athletes work toward goals that have become important to them and simply won't let themselves drift too far from their training regimens.

Research shows that runners at the national level train about 4.9 times per week, while runners at local levels train about 3.2 times per week. In other words, athletes who want higher levels of performance must put in the time even though their bodies fight them and beg them to rest more, take it easy, and just plain give them a break. Athletes use coaches, knowledge gained through science, and the support of their families to help them achieve their goals.

Can you see the parallels with your own quest? You need the knowledge in this book and the support of people around you to help you transform your body in accord with your commitment to lose weight forever. *Biology is not destiny.*

STEP 3: Eat to Lose

Many experts used to recommend (and many still do) that to lose weight you just need to cut calories. Some like to say that a calorie is always a calorie. In other words, regardless of what you eat, the key to weight loss is to eat less. But research over the last ten to twenty years has changed this view among those who have studied it carefully. The fact is that a calorie is not always just a calorie. Certain foods create dramatically different risks and others create substantial benefits for those who wish to lose weight and keep it off.

You'll recall that the *3-1-8 Wellspring Plan* includes three simple behavioral goals, one of which is eat no fat (aim for zero fat grams, accept < 20g). For successful weight control, this very low-fat goal has the greatest and most important impact of all of the recommendations about diet. However, six other dietary recommendations can also help you feel more comfortable, less hungry, and generally happier with your new way of life. The most critical recommendations appear in bold and the number next to them rates their importance for long-term success, based on my understanding of the science of weight loss: 1= critical, very important to 10 = unimportant.

- **Fat: Eat very little fat** (aim for zero fat grams, accept up to twenty grams per day). Importance = 1
- Sugar: Minimize sugar when snacking. Avoid sugary foods (like candy bars or lollipops) as stand-alone snacks. Importance = 6
- Protein: Eat lean sources of protein frequently throughout the day,

substituting plant for animal sources as much as possible (seventy grams of total protein per day; fewer than forty grams of this from animal protein). Importance = 6

- **Low-Density Foods:** Eat/drink lots of low-fat soups and other foods that are low in "energy density." Importance = 2
- Fiber: Eat at least thirty grams of fiber (non-digestible parts of plant foods) per day. Importance = 7
- Drinks: Eat your calories—don't drink them. Importance = 4
- **Calories:** Maintain calorie consciousness (maximum calories for biggest meal of the day should be eight hundred). Importance = 2

These guidelines provide direction, but good examples can breathe life into this critical part of the *Wellspring Plan*. Take a look, below, at the daily record of Kathy, one of my successful clients. Note the great variety in foods, the tasty combinations, and the fact that she ate some source of protein for every meal. She managed to reach the goals for both low-fat eating (only nine fat grams consumed on the day shown) and for fiber. Kathy didn't have soup on the day shown, but she had vegetarian chili for her evening meal, which is very similar to soup in that it has a low energy density. Energy density pertains to how filling a food is compared to the number of calories and amount of water it contains. Foods with low energy density are those that have relatively few calories per serving and relatively high water content. Examples include fruits, vegetables, and soups. Could you see yourself living with these types of foods? Kathy really enjoys the foods she eats, and that is another critical component of the *Wellspring Plan*.

KATHY

Kathy is a happily married woman in her late forties with two small children. She's a nurse who works thirty-six hours per week, in three twelve-hour shifts. Kathy's long-standing weight problem had begun taking a serious toll on her health and self-esteem. She weighed 202 pounds at five feet four inches and had developed sleep apnea, a respiratory problem causing her to snore loudly and stop breathing many times each night. She was using a machine with an oxygen mask (called a CPAP) at night to allow her to sleep restfully. Of course, between the snoring and the CPAP, she and her husband Jim were no longer as close as either wanted to be at night.

Kathy lost sixty pounds and has maintained that loss for almost twelve years at this writing. She breathes normally, without the CPAP, at night—a fact for which she reports gratitude (as does Jim) every day. The following was a typical day for her during her weight loss phase:

TIME	FOOD	FAT (G)	FIBER (G)
7:30 A.M.	1 cup toasted oat cereal & skim milk, 3 large strawberries, 1 slice rye toast with jam	3.5	6
10:00 A.M.	1 apple, 2 carrots	5	10
12:30 P.M.	1 sweetpotato[2] with honey mustard, vanilla yogurt with ¼ cup blueberries, ½ cup red grapes, 20 sugar snap peas	0	8
4:10 P.M.	1 pear, 10 snap peas	0.5	7
6:30 P.M.	1½ cups of veggie chili, whole wheat roll, salad with fat-free blue cheese dressing and 2 tablespoons crumbled fat-free feta cheese	3	14
10:00 P.M.	Low-fat ice cream sandwich	1.5	0
Totals:		**13.5 grams**	**45 grams**

[2] North Carolina (the state that leads the nation in sweetpotato production) has a group called the North Carolina Sweetpotato Commission which suggests using one word for sweetpotato instead of "sweet potato" to "avoid confusing them with potatoes. Potatoes are tubers, which are underground stems. Sweetpotatoes are actually roots" (from *SweetPotatoes: The World's Vegetable Champ!* by North Carolina Sweetpotato Commission, 2002).

STEP 4: Find Lovable Foods that Love You Back

Having worked with thousands of weight controllers over the years, I have come to the conclusion it's not enough just to eat right; it's important for you to eat well. Eating well means eating for enjoyment, comfort, and good feelings. Certainly one of the keys to long-term success is to nurture your love for food, but also to redirect it toward food that can love you back. Find your passion in foods that are constructive, not destructive.

Among the many foods that my clients have found as true examples of highly lovable foods that love them back are the following:

- Sweetpotatoes topped with fruit salsas, cinnamon-flavored apple sauce, vanilla yogurt, honey mustard, or very low-fat soy peanut butter
- Asian stir-fries made without oil and plenty of spices (shrimp or chicken with a wide variety of vegetables and spicy seasonings)
- Asian noodle soups
- Cheeseless pizzas
- Fat-free chili and meatloaf
- Veggie burgers with all the fixings
- Fat-free beans and franks
- Barbecue veggies
- Pork tenderloin, pounded and marinated in a teriyaki sauce, then grilled or baked
- Low-fat soy cheese pizzas
- Tortilla wraps for chicken and vegetables or fat-free beans and fat-free cheese
- Fat-free brownies and pies
- Fat-free frozen yogurt and very low-fat ice cream sandwiches

I hope that you can see how eating well can serve your weight loss goals as well as your comfort and happiness. Restrictive diets cannot do this and are, therefore, doomed to failure.

STEP 5: Move to Lose

Exercise can:

- Improve weight loss
- Improve maintenance of weight loss
- Improve stress management
- Improve the quality of sleep
- Improve digestion
- Enhance self-esteem
- Improve resistance to such illnesses as cancer
- Help you feel energized
- Promote greater endurance
- Build strength

But exercise can't improve weight loss unless you follow the other seven steps in this program. You probably already know that you need to become more active if you are serious about losing weight. The

Wellspring Plan includes just one major recommendation about activity, the second of the three simple behavioral goals:

Take at least 10,000 steps per day. A simple little device called a pedometer, which counts the number of steps you take, can make a gigantic difference in your efforts toward effective lifelong weight control. Pedometers are available on several Web sites, including www.calorieking.com. Research shows that if you can target ten thousand steps per day you will greatly enhance your ability to lose weight and keep it off. Most people walk three to five thousand steps per day (although some studies put this number at closer to eight thousand), measured from the time they wake up until the time they go to bed. Overweight people average far fewer steps than most people (and conversely spend more time sitting and lying down). By more than doubling your usual levels of activity measured by this wonderful little device, you can greatly improve your chances of lowering your blood pressure and improving weight control.

This critical step can help you turn your resistant biology around. Did you know that when you sit down you expend about two calories of energy per minute, whereas if you simply stood up you would increase that energy expenditure by 20%? Start moving around and accumulating steps and you're tripling or quintupling the amount of energy your body burns. Wearing a pedometer helps remind you of the importance of your weight loss goals and helps prompt you to keep moving. If you exercise every day, particularly in the morning, you will increase your commitment for that day, as well.

Though some people can and do lose weight without changing their exercise patterns, study after study shows that maintenance of successful weight control almost always (more than 95% of the time) includes a dramatic change in activity level.

STEP 6: Self-Monitor and Plan Consistently

The third of the three simple behavioral goals in the *Wellspring Plan* captures some of the meaning of healthy obsessions. It concerns the value of self-monitoring—the careful observation and recording of behaviors you wish to change, namely your eating and activity behaviors.

Most experts on helping people lose weight agree on this one thing: self-monitoring is the single most important aspect of effective weight control. The research on this point is amazingly consistent. When weight controllers self-monitor, they can and do lose weight. When they discontinue this kind of clear focusing, they gain weight. One study, for example, found that among weight controllers in a twelve-week program, those who self-monitored consistently lost 64% more weight than the inconsistent self-monitors.

Consistent self-monitoring helps in such a critical way because it allows you to:

- Increase your ability to use *goals*
- Improve your *commitment* to change
- Increase your feelings of *control*
- Improve your understanding of eating and exercising *patterns*
- Improve your information about the *details* of your eating and exercising
- Promote a more *positive mood*

Using a little notebook, you can record the time you eat, the kind and quantity of food you consume (especially the number of fat grams), the number of steps you took during the day, and any specific exercise for that day. Make sure you record a total amount of fat grams consumed at the end of the day so that you can compare it to the goal of twenty fat grams or less. It makes relatively little difference how you record them—in a notebook, on a computer, in a PDA or smart phone, or in your appointment book—as long as you record the specifics of what you are doing every day and compare them with your goals.

When I've asked my clients how often they think about weight loss after beginning my program (with its emphasis on consistent self-monitoring) they usually tell me they think about it one hundred times more than they did before beginning the effort. That's part of a healthy obsession—lots of thought about a targeted problem. Those thoughts can simply allow you to focus; they don't have to be negative or nagging in nature.

PLANNING

You may be someone who lives life rather spontaneously, but most twenty-first-century people use appointment books, PDAs, smart phones, or their computers to plot the directions of their lives. Planning in some detail for situations that might impact your eating and activity levels can help you succeed as a weight controller. For example, consider some of the most common high-risk situations for weight controllers:

- Getting home from work
- Watching television
- Going out to the movies
- Eating meals during the holidays
- Going out to a bar
- Picnics and parties
- Traveling
- Stressful times at work

For many people, such situations produce their greatest deviations from their low-fat eating plans. How do you cope with such situations? Most strategies require some concrete planning, which involves thinking about the situations and envisioning methods of getting through them while staying true to your weight-control goals.

How do you use the following coping responses to manage high-risk situations in your life most effectively?

- Leave the situation
- Call or talk to someone
- Think about the reasons you want to control your weight and the benefits from being thinner
- Exercise
- Eat low-fat alternatives
- Drink water or other very low-calorie or no-calorie liquids
- Use your self-monitoring journal to express your feelings
- Remind yourself of all the negative consequences of being overweight

Research on impulsive and addictive behaviors shows that lapses occur when people avoid making *any* coping responses. Your mission is to have a wide variety of coping responses available for use in every high-risk situation. Having those coping responses well-established in your behavioral repertoire will help you use them more readily when the situation arises. Most important of all, use *some* coping response during those situations. Almost any form of active coping is far, far better than passive acceptance of problematic situations.

I hope you can see how self-monitoring and planning can help you manage your weight. If you don't maintain a healthy obsession, your biology will take over and keep you unhappy and unhealthy.

STEP 7: Understand and Manage Stress—With and Without Food

Imagine starting a day not being able to find your keys. Then you discover that you have run out of milk for your cereal and that the clothes you wanted to wear are not clean. These life situations can be defined as "stressors." Minor everyday stressors are sometimes described in research literature as "hassles." Stress is the negative feelings—frustration, tension, and irritability—that can occur in response to specific stressors.

Your stress responses can be physical, emotional, mental, and interpersonal. Physical reactions could involve fatigue or headaches. Emotional reactions include anxiety, frustration, anger, moodiness, and depression. The mental or cognitive stress responses include forgetfulness and a dulling of the senses. On the interpersonal side, reactions can involve distrust, resentment, and loneliness.

Stress management involves adding control and decreasing the impact of stressors. Coping strategies include some of the ones reviewed in the previous chapter, such as self-monitoring, but they also include *eating*. Eating can produce certain biochemical reactions in your brain that actually resemble many antidepressants, such as Prozac. You know this from your experience at big meals, after which you may feel tired and a pleasant sensation of fullness. In smaller ways, even certain snacks produce the same tranquilizing effects. And contrary to what most authors advise about eating as a coping strategy, I say it's okay! Eating to feel better is simply part of being human. You can eat to cope if you eat lovable foods that love you back. But if you eat high-fat, destructive foods when stressed, you will undermine everything you are trying to do as a successful weight controller.

Cindy, one of my clients whom you will read more about in Chapter 7, lost 263 pounds. She had had lifelong problems with overeating in response to emotional distress, but found that—instead of trying to cope without using food an impossible 100% of the time—she could simply change the way she ate. She could eat when stressed as long as she ate lovable foods that loved her back, such as three pears and a bag of air-popped popcorn. She discovered another key to successful weight control during these controlled binges—that is, *deviate quantitatively, not qualitatively*. You can eat greater quantities of safe, lovable foods when the stress level gets too high and you are unable to cope in other ways. But what you do not want to do, under any circumstance, is to deviate qualitatively by eating high-fat foods.

STEP 8: Use Slump Busters to Overcome Slumps

This book's emphasis on maintaining lovability in your food shows how important pleasure is for lifelong weight control. Masters of weight control do not report suffering every day, but rather report increasing comfort with the process as the years roll by. They do this by making their food special and interesting—and by not allowing their new food choices to negatively affect their personal happiness.

You may think of the traditional romantic candlelit dinner or getaway weekend as requiring rich main courses and creamy desserts, toasted by wonderful wines. You can certainly include all of these elements, including the wine, at a truly romantic restaurant or a fabulous weekend getaway, and still maintain your emphasis on consistent healthful eating and activity. There is nothing inherently more romantic about steak and cheesecake than fresh grilled fish and wonderful seasonal fruit—as long as you still get to smooch between courses of your lovable, low-fat foods.

The recipes in Chapter 11 include dishes that are both delicious to eat and enjoyable to create. Thousands of additional recipes along these lines are available on the Internet. You can have fun and explore an almost infinite variety of all of the factors that make food lovable by taking good care of yourself, much more so than you could by eating destructively.

SLUMPS & SLUMP BUSTERS

Most masters of weight control—people who have lost substantial weight and kept it off for years—report lapses or slumps prior to their major success. Even when they're in their more successful phases, they experience occasional slumps. Your weight loss may slow down or you may gain some weight, and your spirits may find themselves in a similar slump. It is critical to consider some of the major causes of slumps and then understand what you can do to reverse the pattern and get back on track. In Chapter 9, I will consider eight of the most common causes of slumps: lapse versus relapse, injuries and illnesses, scale phobia, permanent vacations, changes in key relationships, work or financial crises, changes in eating environments, and problems with problem-solving. This chapter will show you how to turn small mistakes into major successes.

LAPSES

The biology of excess weight makes it *impossible* for anyone to eat perfectly. Those hungry fat cells and associated hormones make an occasional french fry or doughnut virtually irresistible. Since perfection in eating is impossible, occasional lapses occur for those with very healthy obsessions: *Lapses are inevitable.*

A *lapse* is a temporary problem. A lapse is a temporary detour from the overall plan. Lapsing does not have to lead to relapsing. A *relapse* or *slump* is a full-blown change back into old problematic styles of behavior.

Successful weight controllers persist in the face of the inevitable lapses. They realize that an occasional doughnut or high-fat ice cream cone is simply a problem, not a catastrophe. They view these deviations as acceptable, not earthshaking. Lapses begin becoming relapses when you discontinue critical elements of your *Wellspring Plan.* If you eat four pieces of pizza and consider it a disaster, you may give up monitoring for that day, for that week, or for that year. Or you may decide that you simply cannot maintain your *Wellspring Plan* and might as well quit your health club.

Next Steps

You now have the concepts to help you build a healthy obsession. The eight steps just discussed encourage you to create a lifestyle that puts you in charge of your resistant biology, not vice versa. You do not need to sacrifice your passion for food in order to enjoy a slimmer, healthier you. You can find your own sweetpotatoes (and other lovable foods). The case histories and other details in the remainder of this book will give you additional reasons to believe you can do this, showing you more precisely how thousands of others did it. Just keep turning the pages of this book, get that self-monitoring activated, keep moving, keep eating right, and enjoy a healthier and better life.

Step 1: Make the Decision

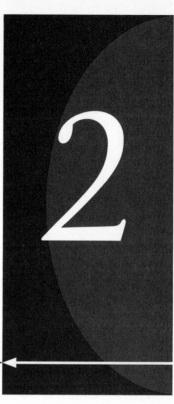

IN THEIR BOOK *Facilitating Treatment Adherence*, Drs. Don Meichenbaum and Dennis Turk describe a remarkable example of how people resist change despite sometimes dire consequences. They described a study by Dr. Patricia Vincent published in *Nursing Research* in 1971 on the serious—but very treatable—eye disease glaucoma. Patients who were diagnosed with glaucoma were told that "they must use eye drops three times per day or they would go blind." Vincent reported that only 42% of these patients used the eye drops frequently enough to avoid permanent damage to their vision. That means the majority of people failed to follow the regimen carefully enough to avoid damage to their eyes. In fact, only 28% of the people who had not adhered adequately to the regimen improved their use of eye drops even after reaching the point of becoming legally blind in one eye!

We resist change mightily. As the illustration below demonstrates, our lives follow certain pathways and constructing a bridge to a different direction takes a great deal of effort. Vincent's study on glaucoma certainly makes this point. Even when their eyesight deteriorated to the point of permanent legal blindness, the majority of people faced with this unfortunate turn of events still didn't follow the necessary steps to keep their eyesight from getting even worse. How, then, are you supposed to develop a healthy obsession that would allow you to grapple effectively with this substantial biological barrier against successful weight loss every day of your life? You're not faced with impending blindness. You must construct a set of habits that makes this issue just as important to you—perhaps even more important—than those people faced with a progressive eye disease.

All Personal Changes Are Challenging

Weight control may pose one of the greatest personal challenges that anyone could face, but all personal changes are challenging. As Figure 2.1 shows, everyone follows certain paths in their lives as a result of many very powerful influences. Your childhood, your genetic makeup, your financial status, and many other factors move you toward walking down a certain road. Getting to a different pathway takes great effort and a little luck. Consider the following statistics cited by Drs. Meichenbaum and Turk in 1987 about the manner in which people change:

FIGURE 2.1: YOUR LIFE

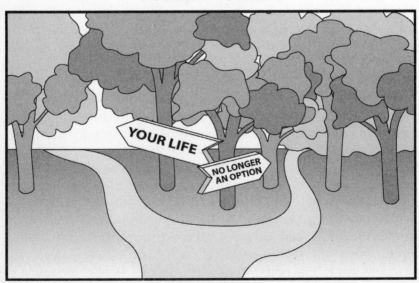

- **Prescriptions.** Approximately one-third of the 750 million new prescriptions written per year in the United States and England are never filled. An additional 300 million of those prescriptions may not be followed in the way they were written.
- **Adolescent cancer.** Approximately 50% of the medications prescribed to adolescents with cancer are not taken as directed.
- **Epilepsy.** Approximately 35% of the drug regimens prescribed for epilepsy are not followed.
- **Pediatric illness.** Parents fail to ensure that their children adhere to medication regimens approximately 50% of the time.
- **Schizophrenia.** Approximately 75% of people diagnosed with schizophrenia discontinue treatment prematurely.
- **Chronic illness among the elderly.** A majority of elderly people who have chronic illnesses do not follow their prescribed and necessary medication regimens.
- **Kidney disease.** Approximately 70% of people with kidney disease fail to follow dietary and fluid restrictions necessary for their comfort and health.
- **High blood pressure.** Only 30% of people with high blood pressure follow the medical regimens that can save their lives.
- **Exercise.** Only 20% of adult Americans exercise at least twice a week for at least thirty minutes. The American College of Sports Medicine recommends that everyone should exercise at least five times per week.
- **Diabetes.** About 7% of diabetic patients adhere to all of the steps considered necessary for good control of this deadly disease.

These statistics startle some people. I've heard questions like, "How could people fail to take medications and follow other steps that are so critical to preserving their health and well-being?" In some ways, this perfectly reasonable question misses the point. The fact is that people usually struggle to maintain regimens of any kind that are different from what they are used to doing. Almost regardless of the consequences, we resist change mightily.

These statistics raise an important issue about weight control. Since most people usually struggle to change their lifestyles, why are obese people blamed so harshly for problems they encounter when trying to make huge changes in their lives? The answer comes from the way people think. People often develop biases about certain topics when they become emotionally involved in them. People become involved in weight control because it is emphasized so much in our culture. They also become involved because they see many people gain and lose weight over and over again. Very few problems, if any, are as visible as weight problems. People often decide that since many people regain the weight they lose, weight loss is impossible. "Since Mary, Jane, and Tim all regained the weight they lost, no one can do it," or so the thinking goes. This is distorted thinking. After all, people tend to resist making changes in all aspects of their lives. Why should weight control be any different?

Weight controllers get an especially large dose of pessimism from others. The distortions in thinking about weight control come, in part, from blaming overweight people for their problems. Both children and adults blame overweight individuals for their excess weight. If someone is an epileptic or diabetic, he or she is considered blameless and unfortunate. People do not understand that powerful biological forces make weight control very challenging; they see excess weight as a product of gluttony and personal inadequacy. Have you heard this gem? "If you are overweight, you must eat too much, and you must be too lazy or too weak to change." Please remember that a healthy obsession makes change possible. Athletes can become highly skilled; diabetics can control all aspects of their disease effectively; people with high blood pressure can control it; children can take their medications as prescribed; and overweight people can become healthier and slimmer. None of these things are easy, but all of them are possible—with the *Wellspring Plan*.

Committing to Change

How committed are you to losing weight? Is it one of the top two or three priorities in your life right now? Or does it fall somewhere much farther down the list? Part of the answer to these questions comes from considering the advantages and disadvantages of attempting to lose weight. When you thoroughly analyze the possible advantages and disadvantages for a particular goal, you become more committed to that goal. Strong, unshakable commitments are critical elements in the *Wellspring Plan*.

The Decision Balance Technique

The "Decision Balance Sheet" below asks you to write out the positive and negative aspects of trying to reach your weight loss goal. First, write in a specific goal for the next year. For example, are you trying to lose twenty, fifty, or one hundred pounds during this next year? When writing out the goal, consider that it works best to state a goal that is difficult but achievable. It is extremely difficult for anybody to lose one hundred pounds in one year, regardless of the methods used. For most people, realistic goals for weight loss include losing between one-quarter of a pound to one pound per week. After stating your goal, write out everything you can think of that would be good or positive about attempting to reach that goal. What effects on your life would reaching that goal have and what would you enjoy about those effects? After writing out the positive side of this decision, consider the negatives as well. Weight control takes time, effort, and money for everyone who seeks it. What are the specific costs to you of attempting to lose weight this year? Spend a few minutes writing out the positives and negatives of attempting to lose weight on the Decision Balance Sheet below.

DECISION BALANCE SHEET

Name: _____ Date: _____

Goal: _____

Positive Aspects of Trying to Reach the Goal and of Reaching the Goal:

1. _____
2. _____
3. _____
4. _____
5. _____
6. _____
7. _____
8. _____
9. _____
10. _____

Negative Aspects of Trying to Reach the Goal and of Reaching the Goal:

1. _____
2. _____
3. _____
4. _____
5. _____
6. _____
7. _____
8. _____
9. _____
10. _____

Jan completed her Decision Balance Sheet in an unusual way. She divided the positive and negative consequences of attempting to lose weight into several categories. You can see that these categories include tangible or material gains and losses to herself and to others. They also include anticipations that are personal or social, not material.

It might be helpful for you to examine Jan's list. After studying it, consider revising your own Decision Balance Sheet. It helps to include all the factors that might result from attempting to lose weight when making a decision as challenging as this one.

JAN'S DECISION BALANCE SHEET

Goal: Lose fifty pounds in one year

Tangible Gains/Losses to Self

Positive Anticipations
1. Improve ability to walk around, shop, bike.
2. Improve tennis game.
3. Increase contact with others.
4. Improve health in long run (live longer!).
5. Increase job opportunities.
6. Be able to buy more stylish clothes.
7. Be able to borrow others' clothes.
8. Go to the beach more.
9. Get presents other than stationery (like clothes).
10. Spend less money on fad diets, specialized diet foods.

Negative Anticipations

1. Takes lots of time to count calories, monitor food.
2. Costs money for group sessions, exercise classes.
3. Exercising may cause injuries.
4. Takes time to keep records and do exercise.
5. Costs money for new clothes.

Tangible Gains/Losses to Others

Positive Anticipations

1. Increase socializing (helping others, being a friend).
2. More energy for family.
3. More willing to do active things with family.
4. More expertise available for family in nutrition, exercise, self-control.
5. More expertise available for friends.
6. May live longer, so I can help my family longer.
7. More healthful foods and lifestyle modeled by me for family.

Negative Anticipations

1. May burden others with need for support.
2. Others in family will have to do more cooking.
3. Will be busier—with exercising and group sessions—so less time for others.
4. There will be fewer "treats" available in the house.
5. There will be less money available for others.

Self-Approval/Disapproval

Positive Anticipations

1. Feel proud.
2. Feel more self-confident.
3. Feel sense of mastery.
4. Feel in control of my body.
5. Understand my body and myself better.

Negative Anticipations

1. Feel too "obsessed."
2. Feel restricted.
3. Become less joyful and spontaneous.
4. Will have bought into cultural pressures to be thin.
5. Feel too much like a "health nut."

Social Approval/Disapproval

Positive Anticipations

1. Friends will congratulate me.
2. Relatives will recognize my strengths.
3. People will see me as a person first and not just as a "fat person."
4. Kids won't laugh at me anymore.
5. Spouse will find me more attractive.
6. Increased attractiveness to others.
7. Friends will like my less depressed, happier disposition.

Negative Anticipations

1. Friends may think my dieting is weird.
2. Friends/relatives may not want me to change.
3. Some people may become jealous of me.
4. When I refuse to eat certain things at dinner parties, hosts will feel hurt.
5. My family may not like my decreased willingness to bake or go out for desserts.

After considering your decision very carefully, determine how committed you are to losing weight. Do your positive anticipations clearly outweigh your negative anticipations? This analysis requires not just a simple count of positive versus negative anticipations; it requires you to study the importance of each item on your list. In Jan's case, improved job opportunities and improved abilities to be active were extremely important to her. As a fifty-four-year-old woman who was more than one hundred pounds overweight, her aching knees and back had become more than minor annoyances. These problems affected her ability to spend time with people who were important to her and to do many things that she wanted to do.

For example, Jan is a high school teacher who loves to travel. During her long summer vacations, she has been unable to travel for the past two years because of complications associated with her weight problem. Traveling was important to both her and her husband. She very much wanted to change this limitation imposed by her weight. She wanted to reverse the aging process that had essentially become accelerated due to her weight problem.

She had become "old before her time." She was functioning as an eighty-year-old, instead of as a fifty-four-year-old. Jan's positive anticipations were far more significant to her than all of the negative anticipations. So, when Jan asked herself about her commitment to change, she realized that it was very strong. When you examine your own commitment, consider the degree to which the positive anticipations outweigh the negative ones.

Selecting a Weight Loss Goal

Jan selected a weight loss goal of fifty pounds over the course of the year. She actually needed to lose more weight than that (approximately eighty pounds). Selecting an appropriate goal for weight loss presents its own unique challenges. A wide variety of tables and recommendations exist that could lead to dramatically different goals. I recommend using Table 2.1 below when selecting your goal. This table, from the U.S. Departments of Agriculture and Health and Human Services, presents a wide range of desirable weights for people in two different age categories: nineteen to thirty-four and thirty-five and older.

	Weight in pounds	
Height	19 to 34 years	35 years and over
5'0"	97–128	108–138
5'1"	101–132	111–143
5'2"	104–137	115–148
5'3"	107–141	119–152
5'4"	111–146	122–157
5'5"	114–150	126–162
5'6"	118–155	130–167
5'7"	121–160	134–172
5'8"	125–164	138–178
5'9"	129–169	142–183
5'10"	132–174	146–188
5'11"	136–179	151–194
6'0"	140–184	155–199
6'1"	144–189	159–205
6'2"	148–195	164–210
6'3"	152–200	168–216
6'4"	156–205	173–222
6'5"	160–211	177–228
6'6"	164–216	182–234

**TABLE 2.1
SUGGESTED WEIGHTS FOR ADULTS**

The weights listed are based on heights measured without shoes and weights measured without clothes.

You'll notice that this is perhaps the first "Suggested Weights" table you have ever seen that does not distinguish between men and women. This table is based strictly on research showing which weights associated with which heights predicted good health in the long run. It turned out that sex did *not* predict health in this research. That is, for a five-foot-four-inch woman, you will note that the weight range of 111 to 146 pounds is listed. The lower weight ranges are the ones that generally apply to women (who usually have less muscle and less-dense bones). A reasonable goal for a five-foot-four-inch woman is a weight somewhere near the lower end of the range listed for her height and age. If this woman were forty-two years old, for example, she might select 130 pounds as a reasonable goal. This goal is higher than the cultural ideal, but is associated with good health and may be more attainable than the lower and more questionable weights that many people would select on their own.

This table also shows that as we get older, higher weights are more typical and perfectly acceptable. As people age, their metabolic rates slow down and they tend to increase fat and lose some muscle and bone. This results in higher overall weights. If you remain physically fit, you can actually benefit from having a few extra pounds on your body. Having a few extra rather than a few too little pounds aids recovery from surgeries, heart attacks and other traumas. Since older people tend to experience more of such traumas, somewhat higher weights produce better health outcomes overall for those individuals.

Another aspect of weight loss goals is illustrated in the following chart. Note that the "average person" tends to gain a pound or so per year. Some research suggests that many overweight people gain several pounds per year. When you select a weight loss goal and plan to get there and stay there for years, you are bucking the trend. The "you" line on the chart shows that your goal is ambitious. Overweight people tend to gain weight over time—that's normal. It will take consistent effort to become supernormal—to become a successful weight controller—a "trend bucker."

Reaffirming Your Commitment

Your Decision Balance Sheet can and should remain an active part of the weight control process. Review these lists over and over again as you attempt to lose weight. They serve as reminders of what really

CHART 2.1: WEIGHT CHANGE

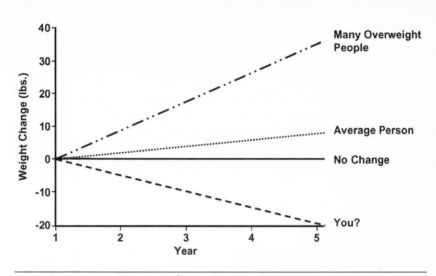

Most overweight and formerly overweight people gain weight over time. When you set a goal to lose a substantial amount of weight, you can see that reaching your goal would be uncommon (but certainly not impossible).

matters to you when the going gets rough. And the going always gets rough as you develop and refine your persistence at weight control. Everyone suffers setbacks. Those who succeed find ways of revitalizing their commitments and thereby persisting. If you remember this and continually refer to your Decision Balance Sheet, you can revitalize your own efforts when you need to intensify your commitment. An important aspect of the *Wellspring Plan* is finding your own method of keeping your focus strong. For example, Jan cut out magazine pictures of Spain and Israel from travel magazines. She kept these on her refrigerator and in her office. They were gentle reminders about what she was trying to accomplish. She also concentrated on the movement of people around her. She noticed how easy it was for them to simply get up and go when they wanted to. This type of concentration had escaped her as she was gaining more weight and becoming more and more immobilized. Now, she could look at people's movement and use it as an inspiration for her own commitment to persistence.

Premacking

Jan used another technique called "premacking" to help improve commitment. Named for psychologist Dr. David Premack, the method involves reinforcing an unlikely behavior by pairing it with a likely behavior. Jan wrote several keywords that were important to her, like the ones shown here, on the back of a business card and placed the card in her wallet.

Walking	Clothes
Self-confidence	Health
Mastery	Energy
Person first	Looks

Reviewing these words was Jan's "unlikely behavior." Every time she took money out of her wallet (a common or "very likely" behavior), she also took a few seconds to review the card and to reflect on the importance of weight control in her life by reviewing these points. For example, she affirmed how much she wanted others to consider her a "person first" instead of a "fat person first." Jan also wanted to feel more confident, develop mastery over this problem that had plagued her for a lifetime, and wear more interesting and attractive clothes. It just takes a few seconds to review these important goals. Your *Wellspring Plan* will come from many small efforts like this one.

Great Expectations

Commitment can get you moving effectively toward your goals. After making an initial commitment to change, though, your beliefs about what you can and will change (your expectations) are what can keep you going or derail you.

If you expect to succeed, you really might; if you expect to fail, you probably won't succeed. These assertions are surprisingly accurate. Psychologists have studied the power of positive thinking for more than sixty years, and while it alone cannot get you to walk an hour a day or order fruit instead of cheesecake, believing in the possibility of positive change works much better than pessimism.

The following examples illustrate that improving expectations can change pain to pleasure, increase motivation and perhaps decrease illness. As you read these, consider the benefits of improving your expectations for long-term success in weight control.

MIND OVER TACO

"I always liked Mexican food, but I didn't like hot spicy food; in fact, I found the experience painful. Even a radish made me feel uncomfortable. I coped with this dilemma by frequenting Tex-Mex restaurants only in the gringo neighborhoods of Los Angeles, ordering just the safe foods—burritos, tostados, cheese enchiladas, and frijoles. The hot sauce sat safely at the end of the table, untouched.

"[A few remarkable things changed my interest in spicy foods forever. During a recent trip to a local Mexican eatery I realized that] when you take your first bite of a hot dish, there is a short period of time during which you can taste the flavor of the food, before it is eclipsed by the fiery sensation of the spice. During that brief delay, the delicious flavor of the guacamole taco came through. But then came the pain—excruciating pain! A familiar searing sensation spread through my mouth and my eyes began to water.

"Normally at that point, I would swallow the offending substance as quickly as possible and grope for a glass of water. But that afternoon, I did not. A sudden insight had occurred to me. Recalling the marvelous flavor that the pain had obscured and seeing the expressions of pleasure on the faces of my friends, I thought: *Why am I experiencing pain while they are experiencing pleasure? The tacos are the same, and there is nothing physically different between them and me. We have the same kinds of taste buds, the same type of pain receptors. It's not fair! I too should be able to enjoy a guacamole taco.*

"I decided to try to experience exactly what my friends were experiencing by changing my expectations from 'pain' to 'pleasure.' So I did not swallow as quickly, nor did I reach for a glass of water. Instead, I chewed slowly. I rolled the food around in my mouth. I savored it. The taco still tasted spicy, but the spiciness was no longer painful. It began to feel pleasant and finally, wonderful.

"From that day on, my experience of spicy food has been different; it is no longer painful. When it is good and spicy, it is spicy and good."

—Psychologist Irving Kirsch (1990)

MIND OVER MUSCLE

Twenty-four men were tested for arm strength in a study published in the *Journal of Psychology* in 1972. Subjects were then paired and asked to arm wrestle each other. The researchers arranged the pairs so that one man was clearly stronger than the other. Incorrect information was provided to both wrestlers, so that both opponents expected the objectively weaker man to win. In other words, before actually wrestling, both men believed that the stronger man was actually the weaker man. Ten of the twelve contests (83%) were won by the man who had tested weaker! These results suggest that expectations can even overcome physical strength.

MIND OVER POISON IVY

Thirteen boys were touched on their left arms with leaves that looked like poison ivy. These leaves were harmless, but the boys were told the leaves sometimes caused irritations to the skin. They were touched on their right arms with leaves that they believed were harmless. Actually, these leaves were from a plant that creates a skin rash similar to poison ivy (from a lacquer or wax tree). So, "reality" suggests that none of the boys should have developed any skin reactions on their left arms and that all of them should have had reactions on their right arms (based on the actual qualities of the leaves themselves). Amazingly, all thirteen boys developed a skin reaction to the harmless leaves (on their left arms), while only two reacted to the leaves from the wax tree on their right arms. Here again, expectations overcame "reality."

Expectations about Losing Weight: "I Think I Can."

These examples of the power of expectations apply directly to weight control. What do you expect right now from your efforts at weight control? Are your expectations more like Jane's or Barbara's?

> *Jane*: I really can't imagine living my life on a diet. I think people have to experiment with their eating. I just need to eat burgers and French fries sometimes. I also can't imagine exercising every day or even almost every day. What if I just don't feel like exercising sometimes? I'm not sure if I'm ready to live my life like a nun.
>
> *Barbara*: I would love to learn how to actually enjoy exercising. I have never exercised consistently. I think I can learn to focus on

exercising and find a way to make exercising a part of my life. There are times when I actually seem to prefer eating in the right way, as well. I am hoping and expecting that I can make low-fat eating a part of my daily routine. I don't want to keep fighting it anymore.

If your expectations are more like Jane's than Barbara's, you have a lot of work to do. Jane expects to struggle and seems to resent the process. Barbara expects to change and almost looks forward to the process. Perhaps it would make sense for Jane to talk with people who have become effective weight controllers. She would find that many of them take pride in their abilities to control their eating and exercising. Successful weight controllers also feel good after exercising. Even people who have not overcome weight problems learn to enjoy the way it feels to exercise and the health benefits exercising brings. If Jane talks with committed exercisers and successful weight controllers, she may start to believe she could succeed.

FIGURE 2.2: STAGES OF CHANGE IN SUCCESSFUL WEIGHT CONTROL

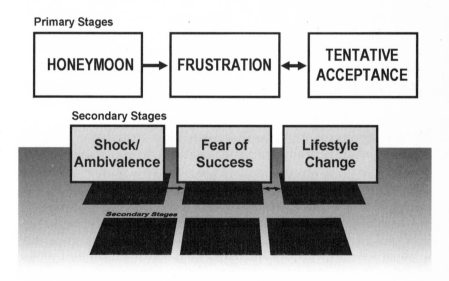

Six stages of change in successful weight control. Based on research by D. Kirschenbaum, M. Fitzgibbon, S. Martino, J. Conviser, E. Rosendahl, and L. Laatsch published in 1992 (Stages of change in successful weight control: A clinically derived model. *Behavior Therapy*, v. 23, pp. 623–635).

Six Stages of Change

What would happen if you expected to lose one hundred pounds in one year and you only lost thirty? What would happen if you expected to remain optimistic and positive when pursuing effective weight control and you found yourself becoming annoyed and frustrated instead? The road to successful weight control is bumpy, so it helps to understand and anticipate the nature of the bumps and how to cope with them. Developing a good understanding of what to expect can improve your commitment and help you appreciate the benefits of the *Wellspring Plan*.

Primary Stages of Weight Control

1. Honeymoon

Thoughts and feelings. Weight controllers in this stage often express delight and a sense of genuine satisfaction. They seem relieved and eager to take control of this difficult problem.

Behaviors. Honeymooners consistently attend weight control sessions (if they're participating in a formal program). They also carefully observe themselves by keeping records of their eating and exercising. They read about weight control and exercise. Honeymooners also talk with other people about health, weight control, and related topics.

Example. Lisa was a thirty-five-year-old nurse who was married and had two young children when I first met her. She had a busy and very fulfilling life. Unfortunately, she broke her leg in several places one day in a serious car accident. That day led to a great deal of pain and a long recovery. Before the accident, Lisa's weight was never what she wanted it to be. It was just on the high side of the normal range. For six months after the accident she struggled to rehabilitate her leg. She went to physical therapy three times a week. She had to cope with the boredom that comes with restricted mobility on the weekends. Lisa gained fifty pounds during that six-month recovery. She described much of her eating as "something to soothe me. It helped me feel less bored and happier—at least for a little while." Eating ice cream and cookies became a means of coping. She realized that her feelings of frustration and boredom led to problematic eating. Unfortunately, she did not find more adaptive methods of coping.

Lisa began participating in a therapy group that I conducted soon after her leg had healed completely. She was annoyed, angry, depressed, and eager to change. She grasped onto the ideas and principles that were discussed in the group. She kept meticulous records of what she ate and when she exercised. Lisa was pursuing persistence at weight control. She was "going for it!" She seemed very committed, dedicated, and happy to have a chance to tame this difficult problem.

Lisa's monitoring of her eating and exercising remained meticulous and complete for about twelve months. She did not resent the effort required for her to achieve a sixty-pound weight loss during that year. She showed remarkable enthusiasm and concentration. Weight loss became a focal point for her. Lisa's attitude and efforts also helped encourage and inspire the rest of the group members.

2. Frustration

Thoughts and feelings. In this stage, people often think about going back to their old ways of eating and exercising. They seem to long for the old days. After all, the old ways are easier and take much less time and energy. People in the Frustration stage resent the effort required for successful weight control. They compare themselves to people who are not overweight and people who have never been overweight. This is a "why me?" stage. "Why do I have to work at this all the time?" "Why can't I take a break from the effort every once in a while?" "Why doesn't my spouse have to suffer with this biology?" In this stage, weight controllers battle life's basic unfairness.

Behaviors. Weight controllers in this stage become less careful about their eating and exercising. They do not monitor their eating and exercising as well as they did in the Honeymoon stage. If they are attending a formal program, they may have more difficulties getting to their meetings and getting there on time. The expression "hanging in there" (sometimes, just barely) describes this phase well.

Example. Lisa, the same woman in the Honeymoon example, eventually reached the Frustration stage. About a year or so after a great deal of hard work, dedication, and effectiveness at weight control, she began struggling. During this stage, she talked about resenting how easy it was for her husband to "eat whatever he wants." Her rate of weight loss slowed and it became more difficult for her to keep accurate records of her eating and exercising. She refused to give up, but her feelings changed from eagerness to frustration. "Why me?" was a consistent theme in Lisa's comments in the group. She could not understand or accept her rate of weight loss either. The year before, if she didn't lose weight during one particular week, she would say, "No problem. It'll happen. I'm on track." In this stage, she said, "I can't believe this! I'm eating practically nothing and look what happens! Nothing!"

3. Tentative Acceptance

Thoughts and feelings. This is a stage in which people settle in for the long haul. They experience a peaceful sense of resolve about weight control. They feel comfortable, with a clear direction for handling their challenging biologies. They also refine their knowledge of nutrition in this stage. Their understanding of the factors that affect weight control becomes clearer, as well. They still struggle with their focusing or commitment, however. This happens quite often when they go on vacations or when their schedules are disrupted by illness or travel.

Behaviors. When weight controllers reach the Tentative Acceptance stage, they have developed very consistent patterns of exercise. They view exercise as either enjoyable or at least acceptable. They no longer see exercise as drudgery, but as something that can help them. So they maintain more positive and effective attitudes toward it.

In this stage, weight controllers consistently monitor their food and exercise. They also assert themselves effectively in restaurants and other social situations regarding food. For example, weight controllers in this stage would not accept a meal ordered "grilled, as dry as possible" if it was served swimming in butter. They would ask their servers to have the fish or chicken prepared again. Weight controllers in the Tentative Acceptance stage do not battle themselves anymore about ordering low-fat, low-calorie meals. They do not feel deprived and frustrated when they ask for their food to be prepared in a healthful way. They feel taken care of and happier when they can get food prepared the way they now "prefer." I put the word "prefer" in quotes very deliberately. Can you really prefer baked potatoes to French fries? Fresh berries to chocolate mousse? Cheeseless pizza to sausage or pepperoni (and cheese, of course) pizza? Most people in this stage might say, "No way! I'll eat the healthier alternatives, but no one can convince me that low-fat tastes better than high-fat. Get real!"

Weight controllers in this stage still struggle with certain situations and still experience exercise and eating lapses (even binges occasionally). Just as disruptions in routines (such as vacations or business travel) alter commitment or focus, these disruptions change behaviors too. Travel and vacations change routines and rules. Snacking during the day, for example, may not occur during a typical work week. During vacations, on the other hand, the opportunities to snack increase and the "I deserve it" rationales re-emerge.

Example. Lisa came out of the Frustration stage and went into the Tentative Acceptance stage. She began to realize that her frustration was getting her nowhere. Sure, her biology was much more difficult to manage than her husband's and other people around her. Who said life was fair? She saw the challenge before her as something that she could accomplish. She realized that she had maintained a substantial weight loss. Even if she never lost another pound, she noted, at least she was not gaining weight anymore. She could now fit into many more of her clothes and felt better about herself. Lisa's feelings shifted from frustration and anger to a calmer, more peaceful state. She still had lots of trouble with vacations and other major disruptions in her routines. During these times she developed a "vacation mentality." This "give myself a break" attitude led to more problematic eating. However, she recovered from these lapses very effectively. She restarted her monitoring of eating and exercising as soon as she got home. She reinforced her own refusal to give up. She could even laugh about her vacation mentality. She realized that her fat cells took no vacations. They remained ever eager to pounce on those extra calories. They loved her vacations!

LIVING WITHIN THE PRIMARY STAGES

The three primary stages of weight control help describe the nature of persistence at weight control over long periods of time. Sometimes things go well and other times the struggle becomes hard to tolerate. After a while, most persistent weight controllers get to Tentative Acceptance or beyond. The double-headed arrow in the picture of the stages of change demonstrates that people sometimes move back and forth between the Frustration and Tentative Acceptance stages. Sometimes they are very accepting of the problem and challenges of weight control; at other times, they become frustrated and annoyed at the whole thing. If they've achieved genuine persistence, they find a way to "hang in there" during Frustration and spend more and more time in Tentative Acceptance. You can expect to experience most of these primary stages in your future as a persistent weight controller.

Secondary Stages of Weight Control

4. Shock and Ambivalence

Thoughts and feelings. Sometimes weight controllers react with surprise and even anger about the nature of the battle that they must face with their own biologies. Persistence is not easy. In American culture people are generally used to getting what they want when they want it. Weight control simply does not work that way. In this secondary stage, weight controllers sometimes become particularly skeptical about the value of working so hard for so long. They seem very disappointed and annoyed. "There must be an easier way of doing this!" describes the key statement in the Shock and Ambivalence stage.

Behaviors. Weight controllers may jump from one approach to another during this stage. They may try one commercial program or another, or join one health club or another, or try a professional program and then drop out of it. The quest for "the quick fix" characterizes this stage.

Example. Ed was a forty-eight-year-old executive in a major corporation when I first met him. He was approximately eighty pounds overweight and had high blood pressure. Ed was married and had two boys whom he loved dearly. He became increasingly concerned about the problems that were associated with his weight. His back frequently "went out" and his doctor was very concerned about his blood pressure. Ed realized that weight loss was critical to his happiness and vitality.

Ed participated in a group that I conducted. He initially seemed enthusiastic and attempted to follow the guidelines in the program. He monitored his food intake and his exercise. He attempted to solve the problems that interfered with eating low-calorie foods and the problems associated with too little activity in his everyday life. After a few weeks of this rather positive "honeymoon," Ed began complaining. "Why can't I lose weight faster?" he would say. Even though he was losing approximately one pound per week, he could not accept that rate of weight loss. He reported losing several pounds per week on previous crash diets. His monitoring became more sporadic and he started missing some group sessions. When he did come to the group, he had numerous excuses and continued to complain about the quality of the program. He eventually discontinued participation in the group. I attempted to reach him several times over the ensuing months. However, Ed did not return my phone calls, nor did he respond to the letter I sent him.

Two years after discontinuing his work in the group, Ed gave me a call. His efforts had not been successful and he was now one hundred pounds overweight. His knees consistently bothered him and his hypertension was barely under control, even with medication. Ed scheduled an appointment to get back to the hard work of persisting at weight control. Unfortunately, he did not show up for his appointment and did not call again at any time during the next two years.

Ed's case illustrates the many challenges of persistence. Staying with the effort required by weight control does not fit comfortably into many people's lives. When people are used to getting things that they want quickly, they have to work very hard to tolerate the frustrations that are a natural part of effective weight control. It is sad when someone like Ed does not succeed. But remember, many athletes do not fulfill their potentials either. These individuals can find other sources of satisfaction in their lives. Most of the wonderfully gifted athletes in this country never get professional contracts, and those who do often do not stay at the top of their games for very long. It is not an immoral or horrible thing to fail to persist at sports or weight control. It takes lots of tolerance for frustration and often help from others to persist. Stay with it and you will be rewarded for the effort. If you do not persist, you have committed no sins. You can find ways of staying happy without this persistence.

5. Fear of Success

Thoughts and feelings. Occasionally—actually very rarely—weight controllers worry about succeeding. They might worry about becoming too small or too sexy. Most people would love to become "too small" or "too sexy." For people in the Fear of Success stage, the thought of these changes produces anxiety and worry. Compliments from others about weight losses or changed appearances can trigger anxiety in some people.

Behaviors. Sometimes people in this stage sabotage their own efforts. They might eat with people who usually eat high-fat foods. They might begin cooking and baking too much. They might put themselves in situations that produce too much eating and not enough exercising. Their monitoring of eating and exercising behaviors may slip and they may begin to gain weight. They often eat in binges.

Example. One of my clients, George, once told me, "If I keep losing weight, I'll get too small. I'm used to being a big guy and a powerful force in meetings and discussions. I don't like the idea of being smaller and less noticeable. I'm just not comfortable with the idea of fitting in better."

Jane expressed a related concern. "I'm not used to men looking at me in a sexual way. Men are now approaching me differently and looking at me differently. I don't like it. I really don't know how to handle this."

These concerns make sense. George was used to being big and noticeable, and he enjoyed certain aspects of his size. Jane, on the other hand, was used to nonsexual relationships with men. She was not used to having sexuality become a factor in her relationships. Both George and Jane learned how to overcome these fears. George and I talked about the fact that his weight loss would not make him a small person: He was still six foot two. He was still big. Also, if he had important things to say, people would still notice him. Instead of being bearlike, he could now focus on being forceful and powerful. Force and power could come from what he was saying, instead of his size.

Jane realized that it was perfectly reasonable to have to adjust to a new way of relating to men. Her adjustment focused on the issue of control. Jane came to realize that she could *decide* when and how to get sexually involved with the men who approached her. Just because someone looked at her or approached her differently, she did not have to act differently. Jane could respond in many ways to these approaches. She began viewing the approaches as positive signs of her improved health and self-esteem. Jane and I also discussed the possibility that she may have kept men at a greater distance when she was overweight to avoid rejection. Men could sense that and would then avoid her. Perhaps now that she felt better about herself, she was more open to a different kind of communication from men. This awareness helped Jane to stay aware of her own ability to control these more sexual approaches. This awareness helped Jane continue to concentrate on weight loss. She persisted at staying healthy. Her binge-eating decreased a lot. She stopped retreating into pints of chocolate ice cream, which was her way of coping with anxiety. Jane began exercising consistently again and losing weight again.

Review Table 2.2 for a more complete presentation of an approach to countering fears of success. This "Counter-Rationalizaton" approach could help you if you are afraid to succeed at losing weight.

TABLE 2.2 COUNTERING FEARS OF SUCCESS		
Fears	**Assumptions**	**Counter-Rationalizations**
I will gain back the weight that I have lost.	I am destined to fail.	Managing weight is a difficult task. Making errors is a part of any learning process. I am still learning to manage my weight, and lapses from time to time are anticipated. I can learn more about myself and successful weight management by learning from my lapses in this process.
I am afraid that others will see me as a failure if I gain the weight back.	I will be judged critically by others even when evidence does not warrant such judgments.	Not everyone is concerned about my weight. Many people can be sympathetic and respect how hard I am trying. Being overly concerned with others' opinions of me is a burden I give myself. I can choose to ignore what others say and appreciate what I learn about myself day to day.
I am worried that even if I lose all the weight, my body won't be the way I want it to be.	I will not get what I want from this process, so why should I try at all?	I don't need to be perfect in order to feel good about my many successes. I can accept the reality that my body is not perfect. I can feel proud of my effort to manage my weight. I can find satisfaction in knowing that every moment of exercise and every pound of weight lost results in decreased risk of illness and disease.
I'm afraid I won't like myself after I've lost the weight.	I will not feel positive about the outcome of this process.	Making arbitrary negative predictions will not benefit me. I am much more than my weight. There are many things I like about myself. I can learn something about myself and feel good about my success and my improved health by staying on track with my weight management plans.
I am afraid that if I spend more time exercising I will feel like the narcissists I have never respected.	People who exercise frequently are overly narcissistic.	I have an obese physiology that resists change. Frequent exercise is the one way I can take care of myself that seems worthwhile and not overly indulgent.
If I lose more weight, it will be too hard to exercise even more and eat even less to maintain the weight loss.	I believe that the consequences of this process will be unbearably burdensome and unmanageable.	Scientific evidence indicates that losing excess fat may not require substantial increases in exercise or decreases in food intake to maintain that loss. Weight loss, however, does require very consistent self-monitoring, low fat intake, and exercise. I can do that.

TABLE 2.2 (CONTINUED)		
Fears	**Assumptions**	**Counter-Rationalizations**
I want to scream when people compliment me.	I feel that others are only concerned with my appearance and not with me as a person. I feel excessive pressure to maintain the weight loss when other people notice it.	I cannot control the attitudes of others. Some people who offer compliments recognize and respect the hard work required to manage weight. I have worked hard to be successful with weight loss and deserve the praise that others offer. I do not have to think of their praise as a burden or pressure. I can decide the extent to which I pressure myself to maintain the weight I lose.
If I lose all the weight, people may think that I have bought into the idea that everyone should be thin in order to be successful.	I believe that my behavior automatically solicits specific judgments by others.	Being overly concerned with the opinion of others is a burden I give myself. My feelings about myself are more important than the opinions of others, which are beyond my control. Learning to manage my weight effectively is one way that I choose to take better care of myself.
I am afraid someone might ask me for a date.	I must go on the date.	I can always say no.
I am afraid someone will see me and want to have sex.	I must have sex.	I can always say no.
I am afraid others will respond to me because I am attractive and not because of who I really am.	I believe that my behavior automatically results in specific judgments by others.	Being overly concerned with the opinion of others is a burden I give myself. My feelings about myself are more important than the opinions of others that are beyond my control. People do respond to each other in part because of perceptions of attractiveness. Those responses, however, will not determine my worth or character.

6. Lifestyle Change

Thoughts and feelings. This stage describes the ultimate goal for weight controllers. Individuals in this difficult-to-reach stage seem *confident, but aggressively self-protective.* They are unwilling—adamantly so—to return to a stage in which they are "mindless" about their eating, exercise, and weight. They carefully observe their eating and exercising. They become very aware of changes in their moods, routines, relationships, work, and anything else that might trigger poor food choices or overeating. They feel confident about their knowledge of weight control; of what works and what does not. Their eating and exercising patterns seem less tied to emotions than they used to be. When eating or exercising problems emerge, they view these lapses as problems to be solved. They do not view problematic eating or exercising as weaknesses in their personalities or as reasons to give up.

Behaviors. Weight controllers in Lifestyle Change carefully monitor their eating and weight. They weigh themselves regularly even if they have a "bad day" or a "bad week." They handle stressful situations directly without using food as a major method of coping. They enjoy eating and find eating calming and relaxing. They occasionally even eat more than they would like to. However, they almost never overeat on high-fat or very sugary foods. They also actively seek healthful eating and exercise opportunities, even when their lives are disrupted by travel, vacations, or illness.

Example. John nearly died about three years ago. He went into a diabetic coma and was revived in the emergency room at a major hospital. John was very overweight and quite unaware of the toll his excess weight took on his body. This dramatic moment helped John stay extremely committed to change. He had a lot to live for in his work, relationships, and all aspects of his life.

John experienced the usual Honeymoon stage, followed by some frustrations. He finally settled into Lifestyle Change after approximately two years. When he got there, he was remarkably strong and focused. His eating and exercising remained consistent and consistently effective, despite frequent traveling and other disruptions. While he occasionally ate more than he wanted to, he never came close to giving up. He would increase his monitoring and rededicate himself to exercise when he found his weight moving up the scale by even two or three pounds. John lost seventy-two pounds and has kept virtually all of the weight off over the past three years.

Sarah also achieved the noteworthy status of the Lifestyle Change stage. She did not have any dramatic health problems or other crises in her life. However, she had been battling weight problems since she was a teenager. After losing approximately thirty pounds during the first year of her effort, Sarah stayed involved in group therapy that was oriented toward weight control. She maintained this involvement for four years, during which time she lapsed occasionally. She went in and out of the Frustration and Tentative Acceptance stages. However, she eventually became a very committed exerciser (after previously "never having sweated in my life"). She now clearly prefers lower-fat and lower-calorie foods. She views deviations from her usual style of eating and exercising as problems, not as horrible catastrophes or crises.

Although John and Sarah had become very successful at weight control, they did not feel in complete control of the problem. They realized that their biologies are relentless and that it takes a consistent effort to maintain substantial weight losses. Neither John nor Sarah reached the exact number on the scale they wanted to reach when they began their weight loss efforts. However, they did get into much healthier weight ranges than those in which they had previously been. They learned to accept the limitations of their bodies. They developed a peaceful sense of resolve regarding persistence as a strategy for weight control. The emphasis here is on peaceful, not necessarily blissful.

Persisting through Challenging Stages

You can see that two of the secondary stages—Shock and Ambivalence and Fear of Success—are troublesome. These stages may reduce persistence or eliminate successful persistence by some individuals. If you find yourself in such a stage, remember you *can* work your way out of it. Some ways of doing this are discussed in Chapter 8, *Understand and Manage Stress—With and Without Food*. For now, please understand that no one develops persistent weight control in a straight line. You may get into a Honeymoon stage that lasts several weeks, several months, or even a year. Problems will emerge along the way. If you really understand that these problems, distractions, and discouraging moments occur for everybody, perhaps you will work harder to get through them and get through them faster.

Are you currently in one of the stages of change? To help you answer this question, let's consider several additional examples. Three individuals—Michael, Susan, and Janet—are described in the following pages. Several time periods are listed on the left side of the page, and descriptions of their behaviors, thoughts, and feelings are presented in the middle of the page. A space is left blank on the right side of the page for you to identify the stage that best fits the descriptions for each of the time periods listed below. My answers are shown at the end of this exercise.

TABLE 2.3 MICHAEL		
Time (months)	**Description**	**Stage**
0-2 months	Michael was incredibly eager to embrace all the ideas presented in his program. He participated in a professionally conducted program designed to help people improve their abilities to focus and to modify their eating and exercising habits. He was a very attentive group member and completed every possible task presented to him on time and in great detail. His self-monitoring was impeccable. He gradually increased his daily exercising from a five-to-ten-minute walk to a forty-five-minute fast walk. He lost one to three pounds almost every week.	
3 months	Quite unexpectedly, Michael began missing group sessions. His eating records became spotty and he began complaining about the demands of the program. He reported substantial binges that began occurring several times per week. Michael discontinued his involvement in the program and did not answer telephone or written correspondence from his group leader.	

TABLE 2.4 SUSAN		
Time (months)	Description	Stage
0-13 months	Susan also participated in a professional weight control program. She was approximately 120 pounds overweight, but was eager to change. She began exercising by walking and occasionally swimming. As she became more fit, she bought a treadmill for use at home. She eventually joined a health club and began lifting weights and stretching with the help of a professional trainer. Her exercising was very consistent and quite extensive. She reported great joy in both exercising and the challenge of the weightlifting. She followed a very low-calorie regimen (approximately 800 calories per day), relying on frozen dinner entrees for most of her lunch and dinner meals. This helped her keep the calorie levels well-controlled. She avoided restaurants and parties and lost weight rapidly. She reported that it seemed "easy."	
14-20 months	Susan suffered a back injury during one of her workouts. This back injury was quickly followed by a serious bout with the flu. These experiences seemed to derail her. Her exercising was slowed down considerably due to the injury and illness. She attempted to re-engage exercising as quickly as possible, but had to yield to her physical limitations. Her eating began to include binges on cookies and other foods that are high in fat and sugar. Her monitoring changed from perfectly consistent to quite inconsistent. She reported great annoyance at the unfairness of her physical maladies.	
21 months and beyond	Susan finally decided this was one aspect of her life that she could control. She reinitiated her monitoring on a consistent basis. Her exercising did not go back to the level it had been during her first year, but she became more consistent and varied her exercising to accommodate her back injury. Susan talked about feeling more committed and more willing to face the problem of her binge-eating "head on."	

	TABLE 2.5 JANET	
Time (months)	Description	Stage
0-1 month	Janet had difficulty monitoring. She understood the rationale for it completely, but, she "didn't want to face it." She avoided talking in her Take Off Pounds Sensibly (TOPS) group. Other TOPS members tried to encourage her to discuss her feelings. Janet resisted. She sometimes arrived at her group late. She didn't seem like she wanted to be there.	
2-9 months	Janet gradually began talking more in the group. Her discussions included emphasizing why weight control was important to her. Her monitoring improved dramatically. She began losing weight consistently.	
10-14 months	Janet took a vacation to Europe. Upon returning, she reported to her group that she "lost her focus completely." She talked about being around other people who didn't have to worry about this problem. She had trouble facing the nature of her biology and the inherent unfairness of it. Her attendance was consistent, but her efforts were not.	
15-20 months	Janet began to complain less and monitor more. Her monitoring improved in quality to where it had been in the earlier part of her first year of this effort. Her exercising became quite consistent. She started talking about how she enjoyed the way she felt after she finished working out. She said it made her feel better all day and much more relaxed.	
21-22 months	Janet's weight loss slowed down considerably. She couldn't understand it. She had more difficulty monitoring. She still maintained her consistent attendance at groups, however. She wished there were some easier way. She began considering some radical alternatives.	
23-24 months	After trying "Fast & Slim" Janet returned to her old methods. She found that her binges seemed to increase as she attempted to stay on the primarily liquid diet. She didn't like the way it made her feel. She got back into a more consistent exercise pattern. She talked about refusing to give up. Janet also began helping other group members cope with their frustrating moments. Janet still had some difficulties when she was sick or when she went to visit her parents. Her food choices were problematic in these circumstances.	

Answers:
Michael: Honeymoon, Shock/Ambivalence
Susan: Honeymoon, Frustration, Tentative Acceptance
Janet: Shock/Ambivalence, Honeymoon, Frustration, Tentative Acceptance, Shock/ Ambivalence, Tentative Acceptance

Chart Your Own Stages of Change

The following chart shows another method of illustrating the stages of change. It charts the percentages of time spent in the primary stages by a "typical" weight controller. This person joined a formal weight-control program conducted by professional therapists. Notice that the Honeymoon stage dominates the first three months. Thereafter, Frustration builds to a steady dosage. Tentative Acceptance emerges during the second half of the year. The blank version of this chart on the next page allows you to enter your own data. Consider writing in the percentage of time you spend in each stage during the next twelve months. You will observe marked changes in your own behaviors, feelings, and thoughts as you work toward permanent change.

This model of stages of change allows you to understand what will happen to you, clarify your expectations, and improve your commitment. You may know, for example, that almost all weight controllers experience a good deal of frustration on the road to success. If you take the necessary steps to grapple with this frustration and get through it, a more peaceful, focused approach is likely to follow. You also know that most people continue to struggle, at least to some degree, with the challenges of weight control. Reaching the ultimate goal (Lifestyle Change) is not necessary for success. Persistence is necessary. As your skills in persistence improve, the struggles get easier. The rest of this book can help you improve those skills.

Toward Successful Weight Control through the Stages of Change

No one learns to master weight control in a straight line. Like Michael, Susan, and Janet, you will experience bumps in the road toward success. You may get into a Honeymoon stage that lasts several weeks, several months, or even a year. During that wonderful time, the process may seem relatively easy. But, as in the cases of Michael, Susan, and Janet, experiencing the Frustration stage is virtually inevitable. The difference between Michael's efforts at weight control versus Susan's and Janet's has to do with persistence. Michael ran into the wall of Frustration and backed off completely from what he had been at-

CHART 2.2: PRIMARY STAGES OF CHANGE

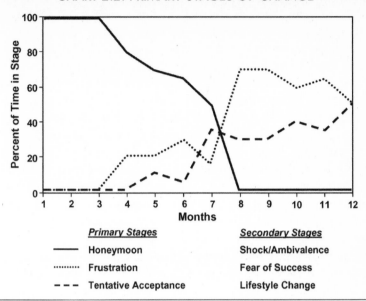

Primary Stages		Secondary Stages
——	Honeymoon	Shock/Ambivalence
··········	Frustration	Fear of Success
– – –	Tentative Acceptance	Lifestyle Change

The percentages of time spent in the primary stages of change by a typical weight controller.

CHART 2.2: PRIMARY STAGES OF CHANGE

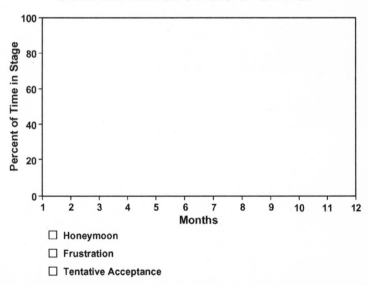

☐ Honeymoon

☐ Frustration

☐ Tentative Acceptance

A blank chart that you can use to plot the stages of change that you experience over the next year.

tempting to do so diligently for several months. In contrast, Susan and Janet maintained their involvement in their efforts and found a way to get through difficult Frustration stages. Getting through Frustration often involves continuing to participate in a structured program of some kind, despite relatively poor progress or some major change in motivation. It also involves continuing to exercise even though the scale does not reflect that kind of effort. In other words, if you find a way to maintain your habits and your focus and absolutely refuse to give up on yourself, you can get through even the most difficult Frustration stage.

On the other side of Frustration you can find Acceptance. Ideally, as you become firmly committed to Acceptance, you will develop an attitude of aggressive self-protectiveness. That means you will maintain your focus despite distractions of settings, situations, and time. If you have this level of Acceptance, you can go on vacations or go over to someone else's house for dinner and handle whatever challenges come your way. You essentially have a peaceful sense of resolve about your body and what it requires to succeed at this incredibly challenging task. As John explained in an earlier case history, "It's my body; that's the way it works." As John felt and hundreds of my clients have experienced over the years, why rail against your own biology? If you can find a way of accepting it and living with it, you can take charge of it in the *Wellspring Plan*. After all, many people face far more difficult and unpleasant aspects of living. Weight control does not place you in a jail cell and demand that you only eat water and gruel. You have a wide range of foods from which to choose. Many of the foods can be quite satisfying and comforting. Why not just accept your particular range of food for what it is, learn to enjoy it, and fully accept the challenges of successful weight control?

The Power of Positive Expectations

Before 1900, patients who sought medical treatment were "purged, puked, poisoned, punctured, cut, cupped, blistered, bled, leeched, heated, frozen, sweated, and shocked," according to Arthur Shapiro's article in *Handbook of Psychotherapy and Behavior Change*. Irving Kirsch, in his book *Changing Expectations*, noted that the "medications" prescribed by physicians in the nineteenth century and earlier included lizard's blood, crocodile dung, pig's teeth, putrid meat, fly specks, frog's sperm, powdered stone, human sweat, worms, spiders, furs, and feathers. These "treatments" have been shown to have no physical properties that could lead to a cure of anything. In fact, some of them could certainly cause harm. Yet, amazingly, some people felt better after such bizarre ministrations! Our great-great-grandparents must have *believed* in these treatments. Modern medicine still relies on the power of such positive expectations. The medicine of yesteryear relied almost exclusively on this power. Consider what you can do if you harness this force for your *Wellspring Plan*.

Step 2: Know the Enemy— Your Biology

3

YOU CAN FIND THE MOST LOVABLE, healthful food on the planet and still fail miserably at weight loss. Weight control is one of the most demanding things a person can do. If you quit smoking, you will never be forced to smoke again. But even if you develop a passion for lovable foods that can love you back, you still have to eat every day and will still find yourself tempted by problematic foods and by the desire to become sedentary or to stop thinking about the whole problem. You can only develop the kind of healthy obsession you need if you really understand your body. This chapter can help you do that. And an understanding of your body, especially if you can really accept your body for what it is, can allow you to make a stronger commitment to successful weight control.

Hunter-Gatherers

Imagine that you were one of the first humans, born about 200,000 B.C. You lived your life with:

FIGURE 3.1: HUNTER-GATHERERS, THEN AND NOW

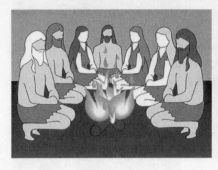
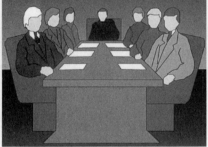

- No refrigerators—no means of storing food of any kind
- No weapons other than primitive spears
- No means of creating clothes other than relying on your own group's ability to skin animals and sew pieces together
- No medicine
- No means of transportation other than your feet
- No means of communication other than your voice

You and your family group would have to spend your days hunting for food, gathering food, preparing food, protecting your children, managing your primitive living conditions, creating and repairing clothes, and otherwise trying to survive, despite your puny physical self. After all, we humans don't have the strength or speed of big cats, the climbing ability and power of the great apes, or the ability to fly like the hawk. Our ancestors' brains and bodies had to work overtime every day to find a way to get to the next day safely. The bodies of these early humans had to survive when the hunting yielded only exhaustion. Often fruits and vegetables and perhaps insects provided the primary foundation of our ancestors' diets, so fat became a rare and precious commodity. The human body therefore developed many safeguards to hang on to every bit of fat. In other words, our hunter-gatherer bodies learned how to resist weight loss aggressively so that our species, physically challenged as we were in 200,000 B.C., could survive.

Humans have lived as hunter-gatherers for 95% of human history. Only in the last ten thousand years did farming develop. And then, in just the past century (very suddenly, from an evolutionary perspective) most people no longer spent their days hunting and gathering or working in the fields. Those in industrialized societies began sitting around more and more. They sat down when they began to work in offices and they enjoyed the luxury of sitting down for most of their days. Unfortunately, though, our hunter-gatherer biologies have not adapted to this luxury as quickly as have societies in general. Our bodies still "think" we are all hunter-gatherers, storing fat efficiently and resisting weight loss aggressively. Also, our bodies were made to move—to move a lot—for most of the day. In societies where people still move around throughout the day (China, for example), weight problems remain very rare. By contrast, our current American culture encourages very sedentary living. A majority of American adults are now overweight at least in part because they don't move around enough.

Why do some Americans remain thin despite our hunter-gatherer biologies and sedentary lifestyles? You undoubtedly know people with a diet and activity level similar to yours who somehow remain slim. Our sedentary culture and abundance of high-fat foods affects some people far more than others. As you'll see in the remainder of this chapter, some people inherit the tendency to gain weight easily, whereas some inherit the tendency to stay slim. That genetic factor and some lifestyle issues (e.g., having a very active versus very sedentary job; living in a household with people who eat high-fat foods versus low-fat foods) certainly affect weight.

It would take a major shift in environmental conditions to turn our fat-hungry biologies into fat-losing biologies. A mere hundred-year-old challenge for some of the world's population is not even a blink in time from an evolutionary perspective. As a weight controller you cannot simply rely on your body to shift toward efficient fat burning. Our hunter-gatherer bodies will, for the foreseeable future, applaud the cookie stores on every street corner, the premium ice creams in every grocery store and the telephones that all too easily program pizza-delivery numbers into the auto-dial. Cell phones, faxes, cable TV, DVDs, e-mail, drive-through drugstores, and other modern conveniences will continue to proliferate, making our sedentary culture even more comfortable, cozy, and inactive.

Your Hunter-Gatherer Body Will Fight Permanent Weight Loss

Consider Mary's frustration with her fat-hungry body:

> I don't get it. Basically I lost forty pounds three times in the last eight years. One time I went on a strict low-fat diet and walked every day. Another time I bought a treadmill and practically burned out the motor

using it so much. Just two years ago I became the soup queen of Chicago. Cabbage, vegetables, clams—every conceivable soup ingredient found its way into my life. I don't remember any huge trauma or specific doughnut or moment of weakness that caused the weight to come back. It seems that if I looked sideways at a piece of pizza, I gained weight. I just don't get it.

Mary's hunter-gatherer body did indeed fight against weight loss every day and refused to give her partial credit for sincere but moderate efforts to maintain those weight losses over eight years. Her husband, on the other hand, was one of those genetically charmed people who wasn't very active and didn't eat very healthfully, but never gained any weight. When Mary worked with me during the past year she learned to use her brain—her commitment, creativity, and persistence to beat her biology into submission. She came to accept that her biology was "unfriendly" while her husband's biology was "extremely generous." *She learned that the journey toward permanent success for weight controllers does not begin with the second step or the third step. It doesn't even begin with the first step. It begins in earnest when all of the steps flow together, relentlessly tightening the noose around the neck of resistant biology.* You will learn how to do that in the *Wellspring Plan*.

Beyond Moderation

Undoubtedly, the most common advice you've ever heard about losing weight is "Everything in moderation." It boils down to chicken-soup ideas like:

- "Don't try to lose weight too fast—you'll put it back on fast if you lose it too fast."
- "Don't exercise too much—you'll hurt yourself" (or "Your body needs to rest").
- "If you deprive yourself too much (especially of your favorite foods), you'll start having all-out binges."

These ideas about moderation sound plausible. Can't you just see your mother or grandmother shaking a finger at you and cajoling you about taking it easy? There's only one problem: they're wrong! Weight control doesn't follow this logical, sensible, middle-of-the-road game plan. Your biology follows its own game plan. The research presented below demonstrates this by showing that rapid weight loss (following a scientific approach, not a crash diet) sometimes produces better long-term results.

If You Want to Lose Weight Permanently, Then Lose Weight Quickly, but Not Crazily

Part of the popular myth about weight loss is that rapidly lost weight *always* returns rapidly. This notion comes in part from our collective sense that crash diets rarely do any good in the long run—which is true. On the other hand, some important research evidence suggests that rapid weight loss can actually help produce better maintenance of weight losses, at least some of the time:

- Dr. Tom Wadden and his colleagues at the University of Pennsylvania studied the effect of weight loss medications combined with instructions on reducing total calorie intake, materials on behavioral strategies, and two different levels of professional support. Twenty-six women who averaged about seventy-five pounds overweight maintained weight losses, on average, of more than thirty pounds at the end of one year. Those who lost the most weight during the first month lost the most weight at all subsequent assessments: Week 18, Week 26, and Week 52.
- In a 1998 study, Dr. Robert Jeffery and his colleagues at the University of Minnesota examined weight losses and psychological effects at 2.5 years in 130 overweight people (69 men, 61 women). These participants received professional cognitive-behavioral weight loss therapy for eighteen months. The researchers divided the participants into three groups based on outcomes at eighteen months. The most successful group at eighteen months maintained weight losses far better than the other participants. Twenty-three percent of those who lost the most weight initially maintained weight losses of at least 10% of initial body weight versus 9% of those in the second group and 2% among those who lost the least weight initially. The initial goals of the biggest losers and their psychological status both initially and at thirty months were similar to those in the other groups.
- An earlier study (1989) by Jeffery and colleagues showed that participants who lost the largest amount of weight initially maintained their superiority at a four-year follow-up.
- Dr. Leonard Epstein of the State University of New York at Buffalo

and his associates, in their extensive 1994 study of family-based treatment for childhood obesity, found that weight loss at five years predicted weight loss at ten years remarkably well.

Participants in all of these studies received professional counseling and focused on a reduced-calorie, lower-fat, and balanced diet, increased exercise, and improved understanding of principles of behavior change that support healthier lifestyles. The people who lost weight most rapidly may have developed stronger and more positive convictions about their abilities to lose weight successfully than their peers who lost weight more slowly, keeping them in the Honeymoon stage for a long period of time. This improved "self-efficacy" ("I know I can, I know I can" type of thinking) promotes better weight loss over time, according to research by Dr. Kevin Hartigan and colleagues published in the *Journal of Counseling Psychology* in 1982.

CONCLUSIONS

Rapid weight loss during a professionally directed course of lifestyle change may prove far more helpful than harmful in the long run. These results do not support crash dieting. They support working diligently in the early stages of a weight loss effort in the context of an approach that has a strong scientific foundation. Driving the weight down rapidly may prove very encouraging, engendering more favorable self-efficacy beliefs and maintaining the Honeymoon stage longer. Then, as the focus and motivation almost inevitably decline somewhat, some degree of weight regain won't have as much of an impact. This means that as you attempt to develop your healthy obsession, remember, especially in the early stages, go for it!

Only Highly Intensive and Consistent Efforts at Weight Control Really Work

The National Weight Control Registry includes responses to surveys by more than two thousand people who have lost, on average, sixty pounds and kept it off for six years. These master weight controllers had lost and regained an average of 270 pounds before their successful effort took hold. Another survey of two hundred masters found that truly successful weight loss effort came only after an average of five previous temporarily successful weight losses. When the masters compared their successful efforts to previous attempts, the biggest difference was that they took a far more *intensive* approach. In fact, the majority of the masters used a much stricter dietary regimen (with minimal fat) and more than 80% reported that they exercised far more than in their previous attempts. They also reported paying much more careful attention to exactly what they ate, their weight, and their exercising during the attempts that led to long-term success.

MASTERS OF WEIGHT CONTROL: MASTERS OF THE WELLSPRING PLAN, NOT MODERATION

These recent studies on the National Weight Control Registry by psychologists at the University of Pittsburgh and the University of Colorado provide important insights about the maintenance of weight loss. These studies involved hundreds of highly successful weight controllers and used two different samples of masters and two different types of research. Remarkably, the conclusions from both studies confirm the absolutely critical role of very consistent exercise, very consistent low-fat eating, and clear and frequent focusing on weight control—even many years after the initial weight loss.

One study included 714 masters who had lost, on average, sixty-six pounds and maintained that loss for nearly six years. The researchers conducted an additional one-year follow-up to determine which of these masters maintained their weight (within five pounds of the previous year) versus those who gained at least five pounds.

Maintainers differed dramatically from gainers. Maintainers weighed themselves frequently and often wrote down their eating and exercise behaviors. They also ate very little fat and kept their activity levels high. Gainers did not weigh themselves or record eating and exercising data as often. They consumed similar amounts of calories, but increased their consumption of calories from fat by two percentage points (from 23.5% to 25.5%). Note that the gainers' level of fat consumption was still, after gaining back more than five pounds, much lower than the average American's (25.5% versus 37%). Very recently, these researchers repeated this study and again found that increasing consumption of fat (and decreased carbohydrates) predicted some weight regain among these masters.

The third study gathered its participants by randomly dialing telephone numbers across the country. The researchers found that the sixty-nine participants who had lost an average of thirty-seven pounds and maintained it for over seven years differed, once again, in consistency of critical weight-control behaviors compared to those who had initially lost similar amounts of weight but regained it. Both maintainers and gainers in this study showed substantial concern about losing weight and much more so than a control group that had not lost weight. Yet the maintainers differed from the gainers in the frequency with which they weighed themselves, the consistency of their very low-fat eating, and their high levels of physical activity (particularly strenuous exercises). For example, 83% of the maintainers reported consuming less than 29% of their calories from fat, compared to 57% of the gainers. More than 50% of the maintainers reported three or more sweat-inducing physical activity episodes each week compared to 31% of the gainers.

The results of these studies show that moderation won't do it. Only extreme levels of focus and consistency (i.e., a healthy obsession) will provide the insurance you really need, guaranteeing that the weight you lose will stay lost.

Who are these masters of weight control? Are they obsessive freaks or only people motivated by impending and very scary medical problems? Reports in the media continually stress that less than 5% of weight controllers actually succeed. But here is the current news: *modern approaches, especially those that use the* Wellspring Plan, *produce far better results than that.* And you don't have to become an obsessed person on the verge of a medical disaster to do it. Recall from Wadden's conclusion that approximately 50% of people treated in the best available modern professional programs lose forty pounds or more, compared with only 1% in 1958. That 50% includes many perfectly reasonable, ordinary, as well as extraordinary, people.

No one who has seen people become masters would suggest that effective weight control is easy. It is demanding and takes genuine commitment and persistence. But thousands of people who have stayed the course have experienced radical changes in their appearance and tremendous health benefit—even reversals in serious heart disease. They have also enjoyed the elation that freedom from this dreadful problem can bring. As Mandy, one of my clients, responded when first discussing the challenges of successful weight control, "As tough as it is to lose weight and keep it off, it is much tougher to live the life of an overweight person." Mandy's success story illustrates that point.

Mandy's Success Story: 236-Pound Weight Loss

Mandy was forty-eight years old, five feet four inches tall, and weighed 356 pounds when she came to me four years ago. Her knees and back routinely caused her pain and her life had become lonely and increasingly limited by her weight. Mandy never felt truly comfortable in her clothes. Everywhere she went, everyone she met, she says, "judged me by my fat first. I really hated that and almost every other part of my existence."

Mandy took to the *Wellspring Plan* very eagerly. She said, "All I wanted was the truth. I learned how to make huge changes in my life and even in the way I experience emotions." For the past four years, Mandy has missed very few days of recording what she ate and totaling the number of fat grams consumed. These numbers shrank from one hundred fat grams per day to the twenty-gram goal suggested in this book. She discovered, after some initial struggles, that "There's always something to eat that really works." Mandy found that she loved sweetpotatoes in many forms, especially baked with "sweet-with-heat mustard" poured all over them. She didn't have to give up loving food; she just changed the type of food that she loved.

Mandy began using a rowing machine that had become a haven for dust bunnies under her bed. At first she could only use it for twenty or thirty seconds at a time. But she gradually increased the duration of the exercise until she could consistently work out for thirty minutes every morning before going to work. She has since added a treadmill, a flat-screen television, and a DVD recorder/player, turning her bedroom into a combination workout room and video arcade. She almost never misses a day of exercise and she seeks out ways of staying active.

Mandy lost 236 pounds in two years. At the time of this writing, she has maintained that weight loss for an additional two years.

Biological Barriers to Weight Loss

My clients have often asked me, "What exactly are these evolutionarily ordained biological forces that won't give me a break?" Let's consider some of the details of these biological barriers to help you appreciate and accept their power. Just remember one critical caveat as you read about them: Biology is not destiny.

Each of the twelve biological factors described below plays some role in making weight control quite challenging. Whenever people develop excess weight (at any point in their lives) their bodies become especially efficient and effective at maintaining higher-than-normal levels of fat. These biological forces include ones with which you are born, others that develop throughout your life, and still others that work to maintain high levels of body fat. Consider the power of the biology of excess weight when reviewing the twelve forces described in the following sections:

1. **It's in the Genes.** Genetic factors are those that are inherited from our parents and prior generations. Mice can be selected for breeding so that fatter mice mate with other fatter mice and leaner mice with other leaner mice; over fifteen to twenty-five generations, this can produce mice pups from the fatter matings with twice as much fat as the pups from the leaner matings. This research shows the tremendous degree to which inheritance of genetic makeup determines the tendency to develop excess fat.

Human parallels include research showing that children born to parents who are both obese are four times more likely to become obese than children born to lean parents. Some recent research on twins also emphasizes the degree to which inheritance plays a role in developing excess weight. The researchers overfed twelve pairs of identical twins for one hundred days. The twins lived in a closed hospital ward and consumed about one thousand calories per day more than their normal intakes. Some pairs of twins gained more than twenty-five pounds during those one hundred days, whereas others who were eating the same amounts gained less than ten pounds. If one member of a twin pair gained a lot of weight, the other member of the pair did also. In addition, the twins who gained more weight tended to gain more of the weight as fat and less of it as lean body tissues (such as muscles or organs). Other studies with twins growing up in separate households showed similar trends: they resembled each other in weight status much more than they did the siblings with whom they grew up. These findings make it clear that some of us are quite likely from day one to struggle with weight control and others are more likely to be lean.

But genetics alone certainly do not determine weight. Your family and environment are also huge factors in weight control. For example, if your colleagues or friends eat high-fat lunches, that places you in a riskier environment. If your spouse exercises very regularly and loves to take walks, then at least that part of your environment supports your exercise program. It becomes obvious that environment influences weight when you look at the fact that overweight people are more likely to have overweight pets than leaner people—and there's definitely no genetic relationship there!

2. Fat Cells = Hungry Baby Sparrows. Beyond genetics, overweight people have many fat cells and other biological factors that encourage them to maintain higher weights. Fat cells are like hungry baby sparrows: both seem to open their mouths wider than their bodies in search of as much food as they can get. Once fat cells develop, they never disappear. Overweight people can have *four times* as many of these hungry creatures as their never-overweight leaner peers (e.g., 100 billion versus 40 billion). Unfortunately, liposuction can only remove a few million of these beasties, barely making a dent in them, because fat is intertwined in our muscles and organs. People can also develop more of these insatiable beasties at any point in their lives. In fact, some research shows that animals that binge-eat (are fed large amounts of high-fat food) can permanently gain excess fat cells within one week. Unfortunately, excess fat cells promote very efficient storage of excess food as fat.

3. Fat Cell Size. Fat cells are the only cells in our bodies that can expand tremendously, seemingly at will. In fact, there's a twenty-thousand-fold difference in volume between the smallest and the largest fat cell. This tremendous elasticity allows the body to store almost unlimited amounts of fat. It seems that fat cells first increase in size as excess foods are stored in them, and then they increase in number. This means that fat cells have two ways to cause problems. Either approach leads to more fat in the body and increased unhappiness.

4. Insulin. The concentration of blood sugar, or glucose, in our bodies is regulated very carefully in people who are not diabetic. The body must maintain this regulation because the brain depends totally on blood sugar for its nutrition and if our brains aren't properly nourished, we can't survive. The regulation operates by a detector in the brain that determines when blood sugar levels are too high or too low. Insulin, which is stored and manufactured in special cells within the pancreas, promotes the ingestion of glucose by our cells.

When people lose weight, the body's fat cells become especially sensitive to insulin. That enables the cells to absorb more nutrients at a faster pace. The muscle cells decrease their sensitivity to insulin, resulting in the redirection of fat to the fat cells. Several studies have shown that some people develop a greater level of insulin sensitivity when they lose weight; these people tend to regain weight very readily. It seems that a great many overweight people are quite sensitive to insulin and can very quickly store excess nutrients as fat partly because of this tendency.

Most overweight people also have excessive amounts of insulin in their bloodstream at all times, which may contribute to the efficiency with which their bodies become sensitive to insulin as they lose weight.

5. Lipoprotein Lipase (LPL). Lipoprotein lipase (LPL) is an enzyme (special chemical agent) produced in many cells. It stays on the walls of very small blood vessels and can become activated to transport fat in the body. During weight loss, increases in LPL occur as the fat cells release their LPL into the bloodstream. By doing so, the fat cells send a message to the brain: "Get more food in us, now!" This means that weight loss may stimulate hunger and help convert food into stored fat. At least for some people, LPL activity seems especially high and probably makes it difficult for them to maintain weight loss.

6. Leptin. Leptin, discovered only in 1994, is a hormone secreted by fat cells that acts as a messenger between the cells and the brain, directing the amount of fat that gets stored in fat cells by affecting appetite. As fat cells shrink during weight loss, leptin is released by those cells. Increasing circulating levels of leptin can increase appetite and in turn cause weight regain.

7. Ghrelin. The hormone ghrelin is one of the strongest appetite stimulants known. It is produced in the stomach—not in the fat cells—which releases more ghrelin as people lose weight. For example, one study found that when weight controllers lost 17% of their body weight, their levels of ghrelin rose by 24%. You may recall, however, that a recent study mentioned in Chapter 1 showed that very low-fat diets do not seem to produce increases in the levels of ghrelin. In addition, weight loss surgery (such as the gastric bypass) decreased ghrelin levels substantially, thereby accounting perhaps for part of the reason these surgeries can help people lose weight.

8. Adiponectin. Adiponectin is a protein secreted by fat cells (like leptin) that helps insulin direct blood sugar from the bloodstream into your body's cells. When the blood sugar goes into the cells it is stored or burned for fuel in those cells. Unfortunately, the more fat cells and larger fat cells you have, the less adiponectin your fat cells secrete. This effect of adiponectin means that overweight people have a greater ability to direct blood sugar into the fat cells rather than using it for energy.

9. Thermic Effect of Food. Whenever we eat something, our bodies must expend some energy to digest that food. Each type of food creates different demands for energy expenditures, or thermic effects. Some research indicates that overweight people may digest their food by expending less energy (1–2 % less) than never-overweight people. If your lean friend eats an apple, her body may require ten calories beyond its normal energy demands to digest that apple. If you are an overweight person and you eat that same apple, your body may require only 9.8 calories to digest the same apple. While these tiny amounts of energy may seem trivial, they can amount to something significant over the course of days, weeks, and years. Imagine the potential benefits if it took you ten times as many calories to digest the same food as other people. This would allow you to eat many more calories while your body worked overtime to handle the food you consumed. Unfortunately, overweight people tend to be too efficient for their own good at digesting food.

10. Adaptive Thermogenesis. The thermic effect of food that favors lean people is part of your body's initial response when you eat something. A more long-term response is adaptive thermogenesis. When you attempt to lose weight and reduce the amount of food you consume, your body has the capability of becoming very efficient. Remember the plight of the hunter-gatherers, whose bodies we share. In order for them to survive, their bodies had to make adjustments when they couldn't catch a deer in a particular week. Adaptive thermogenesis allowed their bodies to survive on fewer calories (greater efficiency) during times when adequate amounts of food simply weren't available. Your body can still make that quick adaptation. When you decrease your food intake by dieting, your body can switch to a more efficient mode. This means that reducing your calorie intake by, say, five hundred calories a day would have no effect on weight loss if your body adapted from its normal mode to the more efficient mode. The good news about adaptive thermogenesis (which is discussed further in the chapter on exercise) is that you can reverse this effect by exercising every day. This exercise effect makes it possible for you to lose weight when you decrease your calorie intake.

11. Stomach Capacity. Recent studies from Columbia University's Obesity Research Center indicate that overweight people's stomachs can hold, on average, approximately four cups of fluid. This capacity decreased by one-quarter or so when the participants in the studies lost twenty pounds.

The reduction to a three-cup stomach approximates that of most people who are not overweight. Interestingly, some people who have significant problems with binge-eating have stomach capacities that may be especially large, even larger than the average overweight person.

A larger stomach probably makes it easier to eat larger meals. It also can increase hunger and appetite specifically for larger meals. The stomach seems to have special stretching sensors that send signals to the brain to quiet the appetite once it is filled. But since the signals may not begin traveling to the brain until the stomach has almost reached its full capacity, the more the stomach can hold, the bigger the meal needed to create a feeling of fullness.

This means that if you can decrease your weight by eating smaller meals (while avoiding binges), you might decrease your stomach's capacity. This should help you feel full faster and partially tame your hungry biology. On the other hand, if you eat some big meals or binge occasionally, your stomach will stay large or get larger, making you hungry more often.

12. Set-point. As you attempt to lose weight, your body uses adaptive thermogenesis to help you become more efficient. Your body also relies on its efficient digestion of food (thermic effect) and its use of various hormones and enzymes (insulin, leptin, LPL), to make it difficult for you to lose weight and keep it off. Fat cells themselves, including their unusual ability to expand in size and number, also contribute to this problem.

The set-point is a way of summarizing all of these effects to make the point that your body will use a variety of biological forces to resist weight loss. Just as leptin has been a recent discovery, undoubtedly there are other biological mechanisms that contribute to your body's desire to maintain an excessive amount of fat. Research with animals has shown that very overweight rats and mice show similar tendencies to defend (or set) the amount of fat in their bodies at a very high level. Part of this defense (or set-point) includes a tendency for your body to respond more dramatically than people who have never had a weight problem to the sight, smell, and even the thought of tempting foods. A study by psychologists William Johnson and Hal Wildman confirmed this by showing that, compared to lean participants, overweight participants showed increased insulin responses not only to the actual sight and smell of bacon and eggs but to the thought of bacon and eggs. This means that overweight people may defend their high weights by over-secreting insulin and digestive enzymes, which would compel them to consume more food in order to decrease the levels of these substances in the bloodstream.

Accepting the Force within You

Now it is time to accept the fact that the biology of excess weight is a real and powerful force in your life and the life of every overweight individual. As a famous diminutive Jedi master once said, "The force is with you." There is no escaping this reality. But you can learn to manage your biological force effectively.

When I explained these biological realities to Joe, one of my clients, he became quite upset, stunned at the power of it all. He said, "I can't believe it! All of my life people, including doctors, told me that my body was basically normal, fat but normal. Now you're telling me that I'm biologically abnormal and that this biology is the main cause of my weight problem? Why did I have to live the last twenty years thinking that I was so pathetic? It's not just me or my personality, right? I really have to live with something that's a physical force within me."

Joe's concerns are very legitimate. And when you think about it, the biology of obesity makes a lot of sense. Why would so many people have so much difficulty maintaining weight losses if biological forces did not oppose such weight losses? Losing weight produces many positive rewards, but relatively brief lapses in concentration (for example, binges and inconsistent exercising) are greeted eagerly by your body's extra billions of fat cells. That's a lot of hungry sparrows to feed! These fat cells and other biological forces are always present, ready to pounce.

Joe had to learn first to accept the powerful role that biology plays in creating and maintaining weight problems. Once he did, he could take some of the blame away from his personality and self-esteem. Joe and the rest of us do not have to overcome our "weak" and "pathetic" personalities. We do not have to go from an abnormal state of gluttony to a normal state of controlled eating. Rather, we must change from a relatively normal state of functioning with an unfortunate biology to a healthy obsession state. Very consistent, very low-fat, low-calorie eating and very frequent exercising are necessary to overcome the biology of obesity. This makes weight control one of the most difficult challenges a person can face.

WE TREAT MELONS BETTER

When I embark on any new romantic or career venture, there is for me always the same bottom line. Namely, I will assume that, no matter what happens, no matter how deeply I fall in love or how successful the project, if anything goes wrong it is because I prefer buttered rolls to bran flakes for breakfast. Or: I don't have fear of intimacy; my date has a fear of flesh.

Okay, maybe I'm exaggerating a little. But the paranoia, the impulse to blame everything on excess tonnage, is undeniably real.

More than anything it's my hope, my fantasy, that someday this horribleness will all go away. Yes, triglycerides are bad and lack of muscle tone on someone so young is horrendous. But so is such a superficial standard for rating human quality. We treat melons with more dignity. At least we wait to make a judgment until we know what's inside.

—Wendy Wasserstein, *Bachelor Girls*

Weight Control Is an Athletic Challenge

Essentially, *weight control is an athletic challenge*. When you succeed as a weight controller, you deserve the same credit and admiration society gives successful athletes. If you do not succeed, you deserve sympathy or at least acceptance. This is the best attitude to take toward yourself. If you make it and become a successful weight controller, you deserve to feel very proud of accomplishing something remarkable. If you decide not to pursue this approach, you are neither bad nor dumb. You are simply a human being exercising your right to choose how to live.

Remember that persistence toward intensity and consistency (i.e., the hallmark of a healthy obsession) makes change possible. Athletes can become highly skilled; most diabetics can control all aspects of their disease effectively; people with high blood pressure can control it. And overweight people can use the *Wellspring Plan* to lose weight permanently. You can learn how to stay in the struggle even when your scale betrays you. None of these things are easy, but all of them are possible—with commitment, knowledge, and persistence.

Step 3:
Eat to Lose

THIS CHAPTER CAN HELP YOU tame those savage little beasts, those extra billions of fat cells that make their presence known to your appetite every day. Thousands of very successful weight controllers have managed to satisfy these hungry sparrow-beasts; you can too.

In this chapter you will discover the seven things that have the greatest effects on your hunger and weight: fat, sugar, protein, energy density, fiber, caloric beverages, and calorie consciousness. You will find the principles of eating that emerge from this review much more sensible, but a bit more challenging than the ones below:

TOP 10 RULES FOR EASIER WEIGHT CONTROL . . . IN A SANER, FAIRER WORLD

10. Food consumed for medicinal purposes doesn't have any calories. This includes throat lozenges, cough drops, chicken noodle soup and anything else bought in a Jewish deli.

9. Using sugar substitutes in coffee entitles you to a free dessert every once in a while. Every once in a while includes two Fridays on either side of your birthday and every Saturday night except for the second Saturday in February.

8. Snacks consumed after midnight don't count because "it could have been a dream, anyway."

7. Pieces of cookies, bagels, and cheese (not cubes or slices) have no calories. The process of breaking the pieces off uses more calories than the pieces contain.

6. If you drink a diet soda with pretzels or low-fat popcorn, the pretzels and popcorn have no calories. The pretzels and popcorn are healthy snacks, anyway, and any calories they have are canceled by the diet soda.

5. If you eat with someone else, the calories you consume don't count if you eat less than they do.

4. Foods that have the same color have the same number of calories—for example, tomato sauce and cherry pie, yogurt and cheesecake.

3. Tasting food while preparing it is not really eating. Licking peanut butter off the knife while making a sandwich for your son or daughter is necessary to ensure the quality of the peanut butter and, therefore, no calories are consumed during this important parental task.

2. If you eat something very quickly and/or if no one sees you eat it, it has no calories. Maybe it never happened?

1. Snacks eaten at movies or theaters (for example, Milk Duds, buttered popcorn, Tootsie Rolls, chocolate bonbons) have no calories because they are part of the entire entertainment experience.

Wouldn't it be nice if the world worked that way?

The weight control plan that I recommend works best when your overall style of eating is grounded in a healthful approach to food. The "Healthy Eating Basics" described below can help you develop a balanced, healthful foundation to your weight control efforts.

Healthy Eating Basics: The Food Guide Pyramid

To encourage Americans to eat a varied and balanced diet and thereby consume adequate amounts of vitamins, minerals, and fiber, the U.S.

Department of Agriculture officially launched the Food Guide Pyramid in 1992. The pyramid presented five food groups, with the grain group (bread, cereal, rice, and pasta) at the base, illustrating that these complex carbohydrates are the foundation of a healthy diet. After four years of preparation that cost $2.4 million, the Department of Agriculture launched the revised pyramid that appears below on April 19, 2005. As you can see, this time the pyramid has retained the five food groups, but now features an image to emphasize the critical role of physical activity. This new pyramid also has an accompanying Web site, www.MyPyramid.gov, which received forty-eight million hits during its first twenty-four hours. This unprecedented interest in a government document was far greater than in any other government document in history—so much so that it temporarily crashed the site.

The new guide actually includes twelve pyramids based on age, gender, and activity level. The site also contains two interactive tools that allow participants to view individualized nutrition and health plans. The first, called My Pyramid Plan, requires entry of age, gender, and amount of physical activity. Then, it suggests how many calories to eat daily for each of the six food groups in the pyramid. For example, the My Pyramid Plan for a forty-year-old man who exercises thirty to sixty minutes a day suggests that he consume 2,600 calories per day. These calories are supposed to include 9 ounces of grains, 3.5 cups of vegetables, 2 cups of fruit, 3 cups of milk, and 6.5 ounces of meat and beans. The second interactive tool is a complex self-monitoring device called My Pyramid Tracker that will be far too cumbersome to use for almost everyone.

You might find it useful to get an overview of what balanced eating would look like for you by plugging in your information and seeing what your "My Pyramid Plan" looks like. Unfortunately for weight controllers, though balanced eating will get you the vitamins you need, it won't help you lose weight. Also, the plan does not specify how to modify your approach to food in order to maximize weight loss and the long-term maintenance of weight loss. That is what you'll find in the *Wellspring Plan*.

Having an overall grasp of healthful, balanced eating provides the foundation for considering the Seven Elements of Eating to Lose. Please review those elements below before beginning to read about the first element: very low-fat eating.

TABLE 4.1: FOOD GUIDE PYRAMID

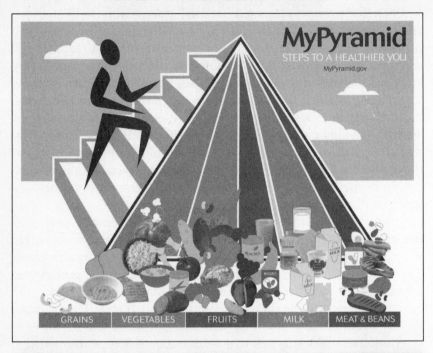

 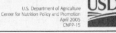

One of the twelve 2005 Food Guide Pyramids (published by the U.S. Department of Agriculture).

Seven Elements of Eating to Lose

All seven of these principles will help you feel more satisfied with your food, less hungry, and will allow you to lose weight as comfortably as possible. The ones listed in boldface type will have the most dramatic and consistent effects on you. The number listed next to them rates their importance for long-term success: 1 = extremely important (very helpful for weight loss) to 10 = not important at all for weight loss.

1. **Fat: Eat very little fat** (aim for zero fat grams per day, accept up to twenty grams per day). Importance = 1
2. Sugar: Minimize sugar when snacking. Avoid sugary foods (like candy bars or lollipops) as stand-alone snacks. Importance = 6
3. Protein: Eat lean sources of protein frequently throughout the day, substituting plant for animal sources as much as possible (seventy grams of total protein per day; fewer than forty grams of this from animal protein). Importance = 6
4. **Low-Density Foods**: Eat or drink lots of low-fat soups and other foods that are low in "energy density." Importance = 2
5. Fiber: Eat at least thirty grams of fiber (non-digestible parts of plant foods) per day. Importance = 7
6. Drinks: Eat your calories—don't drink them. Importance = 4
7. **Calories**: Maintain calorie consciousness (goal for maximum calories at your biggest meal of the day = 800). Importance = 2

Good-bye Fat

"Any pig farmer knows that you can't get pigs fat feeding them wheat; you need corn, which contains more oil," said professor Elliot Danforth. Danforth and his colleague Ethan Sims, both professors at the University of Vermont, study the causes of obesity. Using male prison inmates as subjects, they asked the prisoners to eat large amounts of food and then observed the effects. They found that the prisoners who ate a lot of high-fat foods gained much more weight than those who ate foods that were lower in fat and higher in carbohydrates.

The many facts presented in Step 2 showed that high-fat foods are most easily stored as additional fat in the body. For example, to turn one hundred calories of very high-fat foods like butter or bacon into body fat, your body only expends about three calories of energy. That means that ninety-seven of the one hundred calories end up in your fat cells.

Turning carbohydrates into fat is much more complicated. The body has to change the carbohydrate into a number of other chemical compounds in order to process it. As a result, in order to turn one hundred calories of spaghetti into fat, the body has to expend about twenty-three calories. In other words, it costs very little energy to transform foods that already start out as fat into body fat. Therefore, one hundred calories of spaghetti may translate into seventy-seven calories of fat, whereas one hundred calories of butter transform into ninety-seven calories of fat.

Your biology makes it especially easy for you to gain weight. Why make a bad situation worse by eating fat?

FAT GOAL: HOW LOW CAN YOU GO?

In order to avoid eating fat, you need to know how to measure the amount of fat in your diet. One way to calculate the fat is to determine the percentage of the total calories you consume that come from fat. Certain types of fat (like saturated fats and trans fats) create more cardiovascular health problems than other types of fat (for example, monounsaturated fats, such as olive oil and peanut oil). However, successful weight controllers generally eat so little fat that they needn't worry about which types of fat they consume. From a weight control perspective: *A fat is a fat is a fat*. In other words, all fats contain approximately the same number of calories. And all fats are stored by your body as fat very readily. Studies do show that plant sources of fat (like olive oil or canola oil) pose less danger for your long-term health than animal sources of fat (like butter or lard). In this respect:

1 tablespoon of peanut oil = lard = corn oil = coconut oil = butter =
120 calories & 13.6 fat grams

So, the question of greatest concern to those who want to lose weight is, "How little fat can I get myself to eat?"

To calculate the percentage of your calories that come from fat, first you must know the total number of calories you consume for a particular day. Then you will want to determine the number of fat grams you consumed. You can use simple arithmetic to translate the number of fat grams eaten per day to the percentage of calories consumed that day from fat. Consider the examples presented here:

CHICKEN SANDWICH MEAL

Ingredients	Calories	Fat Grams
Chicken (3 ounces)	142	3
Light wheat bread (2 slices)	80	1
Lettuce (1 leaf)	3	0
Tomato (2 slices)	12	0
Mustard or no-fat mayonnaise (1 teaspoon)	8	0
Apple (1 medium-sized)	80	.5
Diet Coke or iced tea	0	0

Total calories = 325
Total fat grams = 4.5
Number of fat grams x number of calories per gram (9) =
calories from fat: 4.5 x 9 = 40.5 calories

Percentage of calories consumed from fat = calories from fat
divided by total calories: 40.5/325 = 12.5%

MCDONALD'S BIG MAC MEAL

Foods	Calories	Fat Grams
McDonald's Big Mac	572	34
McDonald's fries (small)	222	12
McDonald's chocolate shake	356	10

Total calories = 1,150
Total fat grams = 56
Number of fat grams x number of calories per gram (9) =
calories from fat: 56 x 9 = 504 calories

Percentage of calories consumed from fat = calories from fat
divided by total calories: 504/1,150 = 44%

The McDonald's Big Mac meal certainly outweighs the chicken sand-wich meal in all ways. It includes twelve times as much fat and almost four times the percentage of calories from fat as the chicken sandwich meal. These examples show more than the obvious differences between these choices for lunch. Very few weight controllers choose McDonald's Big Mac meals as the mainstay of their diets. However, this meal, as well as the chicken sandwich meal, illustrate that one way of measuring the amount of fat in your diet requires attention to the number of fat grams consumed and the total number of calories consumed. A good rule of thumb for weight control is to aim for less than 10% of your total daily calories to come from fat.

SPECIFIC FAT GOAL: AS LOW AS YOU CAN GO (AIM FOR 0G OF FAT PER DAY; ACCEPT UP TO 20G PER DAY)

Some recent studies indicate that though obese people might eat a similar number of total calories compared to non-obese people—most often eat 25% more fat. If you want to lose weight, you must consume very low percentages of fat every day. The American Heart Association suggests that if Americans adopted a diet consisting of 30% of calories from fat, heart disease would be much less of a problem than it is right now in this country. Right now Americans currently consume closer to 34% of their total calories from fat. While a diet that receives 30% of its calories from fat might improve the health of some people, this level is still far too high for you and others who wish to lose weight. Some experts recommend that a better percentage for weight controllers is 20%. My recommendation is even simpler than that: consume as low a percentage of your total intake from fat as you can tolerate (and less than 10% if at all possible). So, the answer to the question, How low can you go? is: as low as possible! More specifically, aim for 0g of fat per day and accept up to 20g of fat per day. Not only is this low-fat goal clearer than 10 or 20% of calories from fat, research shows that it works better too.

Living with a very low-fat eating plan does present challenges. This is the age of motorized dessert carts and specialty cookie shops on every street corner. While people talk about exercising more than ever before, who could forget the image of former president Bill Clinton jogging to fast food restaurants? Some enjoy wearing exercise clothes, but actually participating in the exercise is a different story. The same applies to living life without high-fat foods. For example, in a June 2002 *Consumer Reports* article, the editors noted that Americans were "still saying cheese." That is, "Americans have soured on whole milk in the past twenty-five years and now choose low-fat milk more often. But consumption of high-fat cheeses has more than doubled in the same period, and even cream is rising."

Virtually all successful weight controllers consume much less fat in their eating plans than does the average American. This means they rarely eat red meat, hardly ever eat desserts other than fruit or low-fat/

no-fat alternatives, and almost never eat fried foods. Their salad dressings are almost always fat-free, low-fat, or low-calorie and when they order salads in restaurants, salad dressings are ordered on the side. They grill and broil and bake and steam foods and they insist on being served foods prepared similarly in restaurants. Successful weight controllers rarely eat anything with high-fat gravies or sauces. No-fat or low-fat cheeses, ice cream, and mayonnaise are also among their possibilities. They think of normal-fat cookies, brownies, cake, and candy as foods for others, not for themselves.

Many people really *do* live this way (including me). For example, if you have made the change from whole milk to skim milk, do you miss drinking whole milk, or does it seem more like cream to you now? People find some of these changes easier to implement than you might expect. For example, consider the following comments from some of my more successful clients:

- "It's amazing, but I don't even want candy anymore. When I see candy, or people eating candy, I don't have the slightest interest in eating it."
- "I find fried foods disgustingly greasy now. Except for French fries, fried foods don't tempt me in the least. Okay, maybe onion rings tempt me a little, too."
- "This is the best time in history for living with fat-free and low-fat foods. There are so many perfectly good choices."
- "I now think of high-fat foods as 'alien foods.' I say to myself, 'that stuff is for people from other worlds.'"

FAT-FREE EATING TIPS

Some ideas about foods that have helped my clients make low-fat eating more palatable include the fifty-plus wonderful recipes in Chapter 11. Other ideas are:

- Snacks: air-popped popcorn, pretzels, fruit, rice cakes, sugar-free Jell-O, low-calorie cocoa, the usual raw vegetables (pre-peeled mini-carrots and sugar snap peas are especially good).
- Mustard on everything; collect, compare, and contrast many different varieties of mustard.
- Salsa on everything: become a salsa connoisseur and collect, compare, and contrast many different varieties.
- Pasta, pasta, pasta.
- Tomato sauces: particularly low-fat versions.

- Fish, shellfish.
- Stir-fried cooking: use broths and/or water, but no oil if possible.
- No-fat cheeses: try melting them on bagels or English muffins.
- Baked potatoes with dry, 1% cottage cheese or very low-fat yogurt instead of sour cream. Did you know that a medium-sized baked sweetpotato has one hundred fewer calories than a medium-sized baked potato (118 versus 220)?
- Soups: experiment with vegetables, beans, bones.
- Frozen entrées that specify amount and percent of fat (limit to 20% of total calories). Examples with 10% of calories from fat or less: Healthy Choice ravioli, Healthy Choice linguini with shrimp, Tyson roasted chicken, and Ultra Slim-Fast mesquite chicken.
- Canned no-fat soups.
- Baked goods made with fruit purées instead of oil and shortening.
- Marinades made of fat-free broths—not oils.
- Fish that has been wrapped in lettuce before baking to retain moisture. (Remove lettuce before serving—unless, of course, you love the taste of soggy, fishy lettuce!)
- Yogurt or evaporated skim milk or cottage cheese instead of cream.
- Vegetable purées in sauces. Mashed or puréed potatoes make a good thickener.
- Two egg whites instead of one whole egg.
- Vegetables or pastas in meat dishes to decrease the amount of meat (and fat) per serving.

Nearly fat-free eating is very possible and very tasty. On the other hand, berries do not quite match the taste sensations of cheesecakes or chocolate mousses. Grilled swordfish may be a real treat, but it does not taste like a porterhouse steak. Unfortunately, high-fat food choices must become "alien food" to you, if you expect to lose weight and keep it off forever. You *can* do it. Many, many thousands of people have made the switch to very low-fat eating. It becomes a way of life and can be very satisfying.

The following fat facts, some of which have just been reviewed in this chapter, underscore my emphasis on mastering this aspect of eating in order to lose weight and keep it off. Please review them carefully. If you know your enemy well (fat, in this case), you can defeat it more readily.

- Your body uses very little energy to digest and store high-fat foods (for example, three calories of energy are expended to digest one hundred calories of bacon); your body uses much more energy to

digest carbohydrates (twenty-two calories expended to digest one hundred calories of pasta).
- When you eat high-fat foods, the fat goes into storage very quickly—into your billions of hungry extra fat cells. When a never-overweight person eats high-fat foods, the fat goes into the muscles to be used as fuel.
- High-fat foods can cause an increase in appetite for more high-fat foods.
- Highly successful weight controllers report that their current successes, unlike prior weight losses, became permanent when they learned to eat very little fat.
- Goal for fat intake per day: as low as you can go; you only need three to five fat grams per day for nutritional health.

The following case provides an excellent example of how one of my clients focused her weight loss efforts on *very* low-fat eating. This focus led to great consistency and very satisfying long-term results.

CONNIE'S PERMANENT TWENTY-POUND WEIGHT LOSS:
"IT'S MY BODY; THAT'S THE WAY IT WORKS."

Connie was sixty-one when we first met three years ago. She owns a successful, but very stressful, small business with twenty-seven employees and is happily married to her second husband, who is in a similar line of work. She lived primarily in Chicago, but spent a lot of time commuting to a distant suburb, where her ex-husband and their two grown daughters lived. She also did considerable traveling for work. In fact, she estimated that she ate approximately one-third of her meals at restaurants.

Connie was quite happy in her work and with her marriage (seven years at the time of our initial meeting). However, she was very dissatisfied with her weight and fitness levels. She had been used to living her life as a trim, five-foot-four-inch, 130-pound woman who was fairly athletic. Over the past ten years, however, as life had become more complex with more commuting and less available time, her exercising became more sporadic and her weight increased by twenty-four pounds. Although she was not substantially overweight and the health risks of this amount of excess weight were modest, it really bothered her a great deal to feel as though she was in a body that, as she said, "wasn't right for me."

Connie's main barriers to successful and permanent weight control were:

- Inconsistent exercise and sedentary living.
- Excessive drinking (one or two glasses of wine, sometimes much more every week or two).
- Often minimal eating early in the day or midday, with excessive eating in the evening.
- Some variability in consumption of fat (e.g., regular salad dressings on salads; bar food fairly often).

Connie had one perfect tendency for a weight controller: she liked looking at the details of her life. She was not at all adverse to monitoring, measuring, and focusing on exactly what she ate, how she moved, and the circumstances that affected her both positively and negatively. She and I used this tendency to her advantage by encouraging her to use her PDA to keep careful track of her eating and exercising. She did this religiously and enjoyed the process. She also began incorporating a more consistent eating pattern, beginning with breakfast in the morning and then a modest lunch. She loved and sought out vegetable sandwiches, essentially salads between two slices of bread, usually with mustard as a condiment.

Connie and I did not focus directly on decreasing her drinking, even though it might be a problem. She didn't want to modify her drinking and believed she could incorporate it at a moderate level into a healthy lifestyle.

The following food records were obtained approximately six months after Connie started her program with me. She had already lost all twenty-four pounds by the time this example of her food record began. So, these records indicate what sort of diet worked for Connie (and still works for her three years after beginning this effort). You will note in these records that she ate very limited amounts of fat. She and I both saw that as a critical aspect of her success. What does not appear in these records, but was included in Connie's actual daily records, was her exercising. This included at least thirty minutes of exercise virtually every single day—generally walking, running, using a treadmill, some strength training, and various stretching and related exercises.

Take a look at these food records and consider what elements of Connie's approach you might incorporate into your own patterns. For example, you may wish to avoid using your calories for alcohol the way Connie does, but you might follow her example in minimizing your consumption of fat whenever and wherever possible.

MONDAY, JANUARY 6 / WEIGHT: 131.0

Time	Food	Calories	Fat Grams
7:00 A.M.	Coffee	25	0.5
	Banana/orange juice shake	165	1.0
Noon	Fruit	200	1.0
7:00 P.M.	Rice	200	0.0
	Shrimp	90	1.0
	Salmon	120	5.0
	Pretzels	100	0.0
	Wine	270	0.0
	Skim milk	90	0.0
	Frozen yogurt	120	0.0
	Totals	**1,380**	**8.5**

TUESDAY, JANUARY 7 / WEIGHT: 130.0

Time	Food	Calories	Fat Grams
7:00 A.M.	Coffee	25	0.5
	Cereal	140	0.0
Noon	Veggie sandwich	180	1.5
	Turkey, 1 slice	20	0.5
8:00 P.M.	Veggies	100	2.0
	Mashed sweetpotatoes	200	1.0
	Rolls	60	0.5
	Pretzels	100	0.0
	Frozen yogurt	120	0.0
	Milk	90	0.0
	Totals	**1,035**	**6.0**

SATURDAY, OCTOBER 11 / WEIGHT: 131.0

Time	Food	Calories	Fat Grams
7:00 A.M.	Cereal	140	0.0
	Coffee	25	0.5
Noon	Veggie sandwich	180	1.5
8:00 P.M.	Salad with clear rice noodles	100	0.0
	Wine	180	0.0
	Pretzels	100	0.0
	Frozen yogurt	120	0.0
	Totals	**845**	**2.0**

Why Don't People Believe
That Very Low-Fat Diets Work Best?

When you really know the facts, very low-fat diets clearly make the most sense. We know that everyone wants to believe that they can eat very high-fat foods (Atkins—low-carb diet) or high-fat foods (South Beach—also a low-carb diet) and still lose weight. Why wouldn't you want to have your cheeseburger (not cake for low-carbers) and eat it, too (without the bun, of course)? Yet, the scientific evidence and experience of all of those who have failed on this approach reveal that low-carb diets simply do not work. Now, let's consider why all former low-carb dieters aren't thoroughly persuaded—yet. Explanations abound for this cultural resistance to very low-fat eating. Understanding these explanations might help you believe more clearly and fully in the dietary truths contained in this book.

Why Don't People Believe That Very Low-Fat Diets Work Best?

- Losing the Forest Because of the Trees
- Capitalism Trumps Science
- Spurious Correlations
- The Dosage Problem: Very Low-Fat Diets Work Better Than Low-Fat or Moderate-Fat Diets

Losing the Forest Because of the Trees

Which of these dietary dilemmas sounds familiar to you?

- Should I eat because I have a certain body type?
- Should I eat because of my blood type?
- Should I avoid certain combinations of foods?
- Should I eat certain things at certain times of day?
- Should I stop eating after 9 o'clock? 8 o'clock?
- Should I eat many small meals each day?
- Should I stop snacking entirely?
- Should I discontinue eating anything with sugar?

The sheer number of recommendations about dieting could overwhelm anyone. Some of these recommendations actually conflict with each other (e.g., eat many small meals versus don't snack at all). Research Capsule 4-1 makes the point that most people seem very confused about basic nutrition for several complex reasons. So, how do you know who to follow to escape this dense forest of misinformation?

RESEARCH CAPSULE 4.1

Confused about Diets and Nutrition?
You Have Company—Plenty of Company*

- Which has more calories?
  - One ounce of chocolate OR five ounces of bread?
  - One teaspoon of ice cream (premium, high-fat type) OR one pint of cottage cheese?
  - One teaspoon of corn oil OR ½ teaspoon of pure animal fat?

Professor Paul Rozin and his colleagues obtained answers to these and other questions about nutrition from 184 college students, 121 physical plant (blue collar) workers, and 81 randomly selected adults. The following graph shows the bases for the correct answers:

CALORIC CONFUSIONS

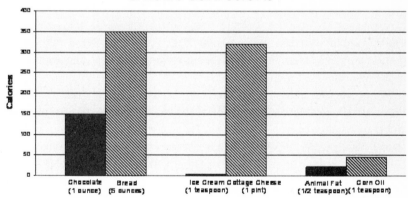

In view of the dramatic differences in calories among the choices shown in the graph, you might think that most people would pick the correct answers. Did you pick them correctly yourself?

The researchers found that the following percentages of people picked the wrong answers:

- Chocolate: 75%
- Ice Cream: 56%
- Animal Fat: 78%

If people had absolutely no idea about the correct answers, then we'd expect 50% correct/incorrect responses, not 75% or 78% incorrect. Clearly most people believe the wrong answers were the right ones. At a time when most adults are either overweight and/or have dieted repeatedly in their lives, why would such seemingly obvious nutritional facts get confused by so many people?

The authors of this study suggested several explanations. First, apparently most of us try to simplify our worlds by viewing things in simple categories, like good or bad. Also, a type of distortion in reasoning accompanies this categorical thinking: the principle of contagion (first described by writers 150 years ago). That is, if we view a food as bad, then we think that even small amounts of that food are tainted or bad, too. The badness of the food apparently is viewed as contaminating all of it.

Categorical thinking leads to thinking in terms of contagion, which in turn makes us insensitive to dosage effects. This means that we often fail to recognize that small amounts of some substances can help us, whereas large amounts cause problems.

Examples of this dose insensitivity abound. For example, our bodies need small amounts of fat in the diet (3–5 grams), whereas 100 grams of fat per day creates serious problems—and even a quarter of that amount is probably too high for effective weight control. In a similar way, small amounts of vitamins improve health, whereas overdoses can kill us. Moderate exercise greatly improves fitness and effectiveness of weight control, but excessive exercise can cause serious injuries.

As you've seen in this chapter, many millions of intelligent people have followed dietary recommendations that are as incorrect as the nutritional choices made by most people in this study. We're obviously quite susceptible to biased thinking (categorical, contagious, dose insensitive) about nutrition and diet. These biases merely reflect a very natural tendency to keep our lives simple and predictable. In this incredibly important arena of health, however, now is the time to adjust those biases. It is time to rely on science to help you decide how to eat and stay healthy. Science clearly tells us that very low-fat eating and lots of movement and exercise contribute to success at lifelong weight control; low-carb dieting does not.

*Rozin, P., Ashmore, M., & Markwith, M. (1996). "Lay American conceptions of nutrition: Dose insensitivity, categorical thinking, contagion, and the monotonic mind." Health Psychology, 15, 438–447.

The pied piper known as *science* can show you the way. Scientists are those who publish in peer-reviewed journals. I've published more than one hundred articles in such journals. These journal articles and those published by thousands of other scientists provide objective information. Such research uses well-defined (and described) methods, accepted statistical tests, and other devices that allow other scientists to accept, reject, or build upon the findings. This work becomes readily available to all, in such journals as *Obesity Research*; *International Journal of Obesity*; *Journal of the American Medical Association*; *Health Psychology*; *American Journal of Clinical Nutrition*; *Behavior Therapy*; and *Annals of Internal Medicine*.

Very few authors of popular books, even those with doctoral degrees, have published anything about weight loss in scientific journals. Drs. Atkins (*The Diet Revolution*), Sears (*The Zone*), Agatston (*The South Beach Diet*), and the Hellers (*Carbohydrate Addicts Diet*) have doctoral degrees, but none have published in peer-reviewed scientific journals about weight loss. They have, collectively, sold tens of millions of books, but they don't qualify as experts on weight loss. Science itself doesn't prescribe one clear simple method for weight loss. Scientists disagree about research evidence. Knowledge gained in research doesn't yield simple answers to complex questions. Yet, the trend in the published science of weight control clearly indicates that very low-fat diets work better than low-carb diets: better health, better weight losses, and better maintenance of weight losses.

Capitalism Trumps Science

We Americans have had our thinking about food dramatically affected by big business. Many billions of dollars have been made by those selling products that clearly increased weight problems in this country. These powerful forces continue to flood the airways and magazines with misinformation, basically communicating the desirability and acceptance of very unhealthy foods and drinks.

In his 2003 exposé *Fat Land*, journalist Greg Critser traced the fattening of America to the aggressive and effective effort of the eighteenth secretary of agriculture, Earl Butz. In the early 1970s, Secretary Butz managed to get governmental regulation of grain sales thoroughly relaxed. This greatly improved the profitability of corn productions and the availability of high fructose corn syrup (HFCS). HFCS, six times sweeter than sugar, enabled prices to be slashed in frozen foods and improved the appearance, shelf life, and availability of high-fat bakery goods (including vending machine pastries). Foods very high in fat and sugar thus became cheaper and omnipresent, contributing to the acceleration of the obesity epidemic worldwide over the past several decades.

Drs. Kelly Brownell and Katherine Horgen of Yale University wrote a remarkable treatise published in 2004, *Food Fight*. In a chapter entitled, "Big Food, Big Money, Big People," they argued very convincingly that huge food and beverage companies used billions in marketing dollars to sell us obesegenic foods and drinks. These companies also entrenched themselves in schools, using substantial financial incentives to create a dependence on them by school administrators all across America. The authors of *Food Fight* supported their claims with extensive documentation:

> At its peak, the 5 A Day fruit and vegetable program from the National Cancer Institute had $2 million for promotion. This is one-fifth the $10 million used annually to advertise Altoids mints. In turn, the Altoids budget is a speck compared to budgets for the big players—$3 billion in 2001 for Coca-Cola and PepsiCo combined just for the United States (p. 6).

Some Celebrities Endorsing Fast Foods (p.125):

o   Michael Jordan – McDonald's, Ball Park Franks
o   Kobe Bryant – McDonald's
o   Donald Trump – McDonald's
o   Serena Williams – McDonald's
o   Shaquille O'Neal – Burger King
o   B. B. King – Burger King
o   Jason Alexander – KFC

Schools receive barely enough payments to cover their costs for each free meal they serve as part of the National School Lunch Program. The à la carte foods (e.g., Papa John's pizza for $2 a slice) and vending machine items yield 50–100% profits (p.146). In another specific example, the recent annual incomes per school in Kentucky were (p.131):

Elementary Schools – $9,215
Middle Schools – $19,156
High Schools – $17,466

The effectiveness of aggressive marketing campaigns like those that sell high-fat and high-sugar items appears all around us. For example, grab any issue of *Consumer Reports* and take a close look. Notice the ratings for cars, laundry detergent, or vacuum cleaners. Some items fare so poorly that any intelligent reader must wonder, "Why would anyone buy that?" For example, people buy thousands of Kirby and Rainbow vacuum cleaners every year. Yet, they cost several times more than ordinary Hoovers and Kenmores that outperform them almost every time. Some people, lots of people actually, also buy cars that break down far more often than less pricey ones that ride better and last longer. An old saying that is supported by current data in *Consumers Reports* captures this phenomenon nicely: "If you can afford one Jaguar, buy two. One you can drive; the other you can keep at the repair shop."

The same marketers who sell overpriced vacuum cleaners and unreliable luxury cars sell obesegenic foods and gimmicky diets. Consumers remain susceptible to believing slick, logical, repeated, catchy pitches. Books with authors who seem credible and charismatic and whose books have appealing titles and premises can sell millions—if marketed aggressively and cleverly. If it gets on TV, it seems, at least, acceptable.

Scientists do their work quietly. We receive no payment for articles published in scientific journals, even in the best journals in the world. Scientists rarely publish books like this one. These "trade books" take considerable time and specialized writing skills. They also demand a willingness (eagerness actually) to do scores of interviews, travel, and other things that take even more time and effort, often with modest payoffs.

You can see why capitalism creates and sells more books than science. Millions get poured into creating and selling trade books, even lousy ones. Billions get spent convincing us that foods that contribute to weight gain are just fine, normal, part of the greatness of our culture. How can objective sciences, gathering dust in obscure journals, compete with that for your attention?

Spurious Correlations

In the late 1800s, some medical authorities believed that riding in trains caused syphilis. This venereal disease had spread widely and caused madness, then a torturous death. Some physicians believed that bouncing on trains must cause this "nervous disease." After all, they asserted, traveling salesmen often get syphilis and priests rarely contract it. The salesmen bounced on lots of trains, whereas priests did not.

Decades later a bacteria was discovered that caused the disease via direct contact, usually during sexual intercourse. Although traveling salesmen did ride trains more than most, they apparently had unprotected sex more than most, as well. Train riding was coincidentally associated with syphilis (a classic spurious or false correlation), but trains didn't cause it.

The authors of the recent spate of low-carb diets have argued that Americans gained lots of weight in the past twenty-five years—just as they became increasingly aware of the desirability of eating less fat. Therefore, they have claimed, low-fat diets cause weight gain by encouraging people to eat too many carbs.

This argument flies in the face of the evidence presented in this chapter. Animals and people gain weight when they increase fat in their diets; when they decrease eating fat substantially, they lose weight most efficiently and effectively.

Awareness of the importance of low-fat eating spuriously correlated with Americans gaining weight. As I mentioned earlier in this chapter, however, just because we Americans increased our awareness of the value of eating less fat didn't result in Americans actually eating less fat. Americans ate about eighty fat grams in 1980 *and* in 2004. That awareness also didn't cause Americans to gain weight. Eating more calories, continuing to eat too much fat, and failing to stay active, among other things, *caused* the weight gain.

Using the before-and-after testimonials to sell something also relies on spurious correlations. Just because your neighbor Mary lost weight when she used a low-carb diet, doesn't mean that the diet caused weight loss. Perhaps Mary significantly increased her workouts just when she started the low-carb diet. Perhaps she started taking medication that decreased her appetite just when she started. Perhaps she consciously decided to eat less (total calories) just when she started. If Mary took any of these steps, then her weight loss was associated (correlated) with beginning a low-carb diet, but not caused by it.

The Dosage Problem: Very Low-Fat Diets Work Better than Low or Moderate Fat Diets

"I had a splitting headache. I took one-half of an aspirin and it did nothing! Aspirin just doesn't work for headaches."

Two aspirins, not half of one, can reduce typical headache pain. In a similar vein, very low-fat eating, but not moderate-fat eating, leads to substantial and well-maintained success in weight control. Most Americans currently consume about one-third of their calories from fat. America will continue to gain weight rapidly, as it has in the last few decades, unless it can change that percentage to about 10% of calories from fat. Many health-oriented groups do not recommend such a stringent standard, partly because they don't think people can do it. But, this only contributes to America's failure to lose weight and keep it off. If you decrease your percent of calories from fat from 34% to 30% (as recommended by the American Heart Association, for example) you won't lose the weight or keep it off. You may as well take a half-aspirin when you have a splitting headache and expect that to work, as well.

The story of one of my friends can illustrate the power of this dosage problem:

Ralph is a fifty-five-year-old successful restaurateur who has been quite athletic throughout his life. Ralph and I play tennis regularly in a doubles game with six other players. Over the years, Ralph gained about fifty pounds. Yet, he can still play doubles tennis quite effectively. He just doesn't move very well, but he has a great serve and good anticipation of his opponents' tactics.

Ralph has talked with me many times about his efforts to lose weight. About two years ago, I gave Ralph a copy of one of my recent books, a calorie/fat gram counter, a method of recording his daily intake in a journal, and a few other tips. Ralph occasionally described his eating program and was attempting to dramatically reduce the amount of fat he consumed. Over a period of a couple of months, Ralph did lose a few pounds. However, as time wore on, Ralph's weight didn't change very much. He claimed, however, to follow the program diligently and to eat virtually no fat very consistently.

At the end of our doubles tennis season, we tennis players and our spouses got together for a celebration dinner. I sat opposite Ralph and enjoyed talking with him, as usual. When the server came around, I was a bit shocked to hear what Ralph ordered. A few minutes later, Ralph's dinner arrived and he looked at it eagerly. It included grilled fish and some vegetables, accompanied by a huge amount of breaded and fried onions shaped into the form of a 5" x 3" x 3" house. Ralph dug into the fried onion box gleefully and even said to me across the table, "Hey Dan, you ought to try this onion house. This place is famous for these babies."

Ralph joyfully ate every morsel of the 100-fat gram fried onion house. He even managed to forget that I was a very strong proponent of eating very little fat and that I wouldn't violate that position regardless of the specialty of the house at any restaurant. I thought to myself, "No wonder Ralph failed to lose weight when claiming to eat very little fat. He ate very little fat only some of the time. At other times, he ate high-fat foods: too much, too often.

Ralph's inconsistency reflects our culture's inconsistent attitude about fat. Some segments on morning talk shows show fat, while others sing the praises of variations on chocolate. The following list of top ten recipes from the *Chicago Tribune* shows no awareness of the health risks of eating fat. The same revered newspaper also routinely prints articles arguing against eating fat. If Ralph were to establish a truly consistent pattern of low-fat eating (good-bye fried onion house), then he'd find himself bucking the trend of "anything goes, sometimes" seen repeatedly in media stories.

CHICAGO TRIBUNE'S "BEST RECIPES OF THE YEAR": STILL NOT TOO GOOD (NUTRITIONALLY)

The *Chicago Tribune* recently released its top ten list of recipes from the entire year. Their list reflects the lack of concern in this country about fat, despite the very considerable scientific evidence that shows the harmful effects of high-fat foods. Review the names of these recipes and note the percentages of calories from fat, even in salads and fish dishes. The average percentage of calories from fat in this top ten list is a whopping 47.4% (< 10% would be ideal):

- Double Wasabi Brisket: 40% calories from fat
- Thai Crab Cakes: 49%
- Chicken Thighs with Onions and Wilted Arugula: 56%
- Mocha Devil's Food Cupcakes: 38%

- Salmon with Orzo, Oranges, and Olives: 38%
- Roast Rack of Pork with Caramelized Maple Onions: 50%
- Fennel Risotto Cakes: 26%
- Yemeni-style Chicken Salad: 55%
- Favorite Things Summer Salad: 65%
- Provencal Veal Chops with Warm Bell-Pepper Slaw: 57%

Successful weight loss and maintenance of weight loss requires consistency. Weight control is not a part-time job. I'm hoping that the contents of this chapter have shown you why low-carb diets didn't work for you and never could. The next step in your quest to become a master of weight control involves developing your *Wellspring Plan*. This plan is clear, easily understood, and can produce the results you've been seeking. Many thousands of people have found this approach highly satisfying and you can, too. Just read the remainder of this book, follow the eight steps, and watch the emergence of your *Wellspring Plan* produce your successful transformation.

Sugar: How Sweet It Is—and Isn't

Happiness is the reward of an active life lived with "sweet reason," according to Aristotle. Writer Susan Cohler makes it clear why Americans often indulge in the sweet part of sweet reason:

> In the harsh light of the suburban ice cream parlor, a gangly adolescent creates a masterpiece. Three scoops of sweet delight nestled side-by-side, enfolded in the arms of a ripe banana. Steaming fudge drapes the ice cream slopes and snakes its way to the depths of the dish. A cloud of whipped cream, bejeweled with nuts and one cherry, crowns the top. This ice cream treat is a work of edible art, but what it does to [you] ... may be worth thinking about. (from *Psychology Today*, 1988)

Sugar clearly permeates our lives. It can provide the foundation to "edible art," and it plays a major part in almost all of our celebrations (especially Valentine's Day, Easter, and Christmas). Think about the well-known phrases "Home sweet home" and "How sweet it is!" Think of many of the most common terms of endearment: sugar, sweetheart, sweetie, honeybunch, sugar plum, and sweet pea. I have personally used many of these terms to refer to my three young children. It makes me smile just to think of them with these phrases in mind, even as I write this sentence. Not only do relationships involve sugar metaphors, but so do our sport performances. Have you seen a sports telecast that did *not* include such phrases as "sweet shot"? Sugar is idealized in these phrases. The best thing you could say about a person is that he or she is sweet.

LOVING SUGAR

Biological roots may help explain this common infatuation with sugar. When we are hungry, sugar provides the quickest antidote. In other words, the sugar you eat is very similar chemically to the primary source of energy in your body—glucose. Sugar is white, refined sucrose that is derived from sugarcane and beets. It is actually composed of glucose and fructose (fruit sugar). These components are readily split apart in the small intestine by the enzyme sucrose.

Several other factors reveal that sugar's appeal has biological roots. First, sweet foods are safe foods. This harkens back to our earlier discussion of hunter-gatherers. Can you think of any examples of wild fruits or berries or vegetables that are sweet but also dangerous to eat? Probably not. If you find something hanging from a tree and it tastes sweet, it is almost certainly safe to eat. On the other hand, sour or bitter fruits or vegetables are much more likely to be poisonous.

Second, when humans or other animals are starving, they consistently show heightened preferences for very sweet foods. This, again, shows the body's natural tendency to satisfy extreme hunger and food deprivation quickly and effectively with sugar.

A third factor that reveals the biological roots of sugar's appeal is the body's way of increasing the craving for sugar. The figure below illustrates one way it does this: when we eat carbohydrates—especially sugar—production of insulin increases. Insulin directs glucose into muscles and other organs. When we eat a sugary snack—a candy bar for example— the body reacts to it by producing an excessive amount of insulin. This probably occurs because the body is programmed to eat large amounts of sugar or sweet foods whenever they are available. This made sense for hunter-gatherers. If they found something that tasted sweet, their bodies wanted to encourage them to eat large quantities of it. So when you eat that candy bar, your body is over prepared to digest it. This over preparedness includes an excess amount of insulin that clears the blood of most of its energy supply (glucose). This results in a very low level of glucose in the blood. The brain then detects this low level of glucose and causes a substantial increase in hunger. In other words, *when you eat sugary foods, it creates a biochemical chain reaction leading to increased hunger.*

FIGURE 4.1: THE SUGAR CYCLE

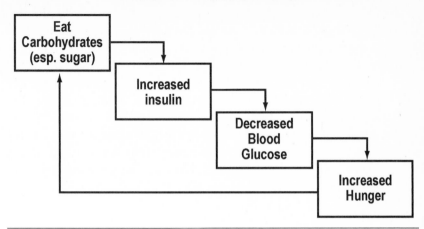

The biochemical chain reaction that contributes to increased hunger after eating sugary foods. Based in part on research by P. Geiselman & D. Novin, published in 1982 (The role of carbohydrates in appetite, hunger and obesity. *Appetite*, v. 3, pp. 203–223).

The research that supports these assertions includes studies in which rabbits were fed glucose directly into their stomachs. These rabbits then ate more, after receiving a high dose of sugar, than they did under normal conditions and quite a bit more than rabbits who received only salt water. I've already discussed how fat begets fat; now you can see how sugar begets more sugar.

Mark, a very dedicated weight controller, tried to eat all the right things. Early on in his participation in my program, I noticed that he ate muesli regularly for breakfast. Muesli, granola, and similar cereals have a reputation of being health foods. After all, they are made from whole grains, contain lots of fiber, and are sold in health food stores. Unfortunately, they contain lots of sugar. Sometimes the sugar is in the form of honey. But your body can't tell the difference between honey and sugar. Honey does contain small amounts of such minerals as potassium and calcium, but you would have to eat two hundred tablespoons of honey to meet the body's daily requirement for calcium.

Eventually, Mark was persuaded that his muesli wasn't great for him. He substituted shredded wheat and was amazed that this simple change resulted in much less hunger throughout the day and dramatically decreased cravings for sweets.

Recently, a new member joined the group in which Mark partici-pated. Linda was eating low-fat granola for breakfast regularly. She also snacked on candy bars later in the morning and sometimes in the after-noon as well. This pattern had contributed to significant weight gain over the past couple of years. Mark and I persuaded Linda to substitute a low-sugar food for her granola. Agreeing that "it's worth a shot," she began eating a bagel and low-fat cream cheese as an alternative to her usual breakfast of granola. She came back from this experiment say-ing, "The 'Muesli Syndrome' lives! I can't believe what a difference this made. I'm also amazed that it worked immediately. As soon as I started eating bagels instead of granola, I didn't have that gnawing feeling in my stomach anymore at ten o'clock. Wow!"

ENERGY BOOST: CANDY VERSUS TEN-MINUTE WALKS

Robert Thayer, a California State University psychologist, conduct-ed an important study demonstrating that sugar can also affect your mood. Thayer compared the effects of eating a half-ounce candy bar (of any type) with taking a rapid ten-minute walk. When subjects took a ten-minute walk, their tension-level ratings over the next two hours decreased very quickly and stayed much lower than they were before taking the walk. In contrast, after they ate the candy bar, tension levels increased over a sixty-minute period and stayed high for the subse-quent hour as well.

Similar effects occurred for ratings of energy levels. Subjects indi-cated feeling more energized for thirty minutes after eating the candy bar, but their energy levels fell to much lower levels one to two hours later. In contrast, when subjects took walks, their energy levels in-creased dramatically during the first thirty minutes and stayed well above their pre-walk states for two hours afterward. Eating candy can cause a groggy or tired feeling because it stimulates the release of a natural tranquilizer in our brains called serotonin.

These findings, summarized in Chart 4.1, are very important. They suggest a good alternative to eating sugary snacks in order to feel ener-gized. A ten-minute brisk walk can provide a much better energy boost than a candy bar. You won't find commercials encouraging people to take ten-minute walks for that "quick energy boost," though you will find plenty of commercials hawking candy bars for that purpose. Now you know the truth about which works better.

CHART 4.1: RATINGS OF ENERGY LEVELS

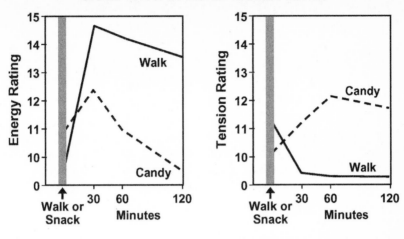

A 10-minute brisk walk can provide a much better energy boost than eating a candy bar. Based on research by R. Thayer, published in 1987 (Energy, tiredness, and tension effects of a sugar snack versus moderate exercise. *Journal of Personality and Social Psychology*, v. 52, pp. 119–125).

CONCLUSION

The moral of this story is: avoid sugary foods and instead take brief walks to reenergize. It is most helpful to avoid eating any snacks that contain lots of sugar, such as candy bars, ice cream cones, granola bars, caramel corn, and cookies. It is also very wise to avoid sugary breakfast cereals. Instead, try low-sugar cereals, bagels, fruit, crackers, or raw vegetables. Some of these sugary foods have tremendous nostalgic appeal. As Gail's story below reveals, changing nostalgia-based food preferences can be very difficult.

GAIL'S CHRISTMAS COOKIE TRADITION

Gail began working with me on a major effort to lose weight six years ago and continues attending weekly group meetings as of this writing. Gail is a forty-two-year-old high school teacher and a dedicated mother of two children. She had gained fifty pounds gradually over twelve years and had two pregnancies during a hectic (but sedentary) life.

Gail became energized during a classic Honeymoon stage when she first came to our group. She monitored her eating and exercising meticulously and focused beautifully. She varied her exercising, starting with slow but consistent walking—experimenting with racquetball and swimming. She modified her eating to include primarily foods that were low in fat and sugar. Gail lapsed occasionally by eating cookies and other sweets, but she took these lapses in stride and kept moving forward persistently.

Then, six months into her Honeymoon, after losing twenty-eight pounds, came Christmas. "I've got to make my cookies!" she reported.

"What do you mean 'got to'? And, how many cookies are you talking about, anyway?" I asked.

"I mean I've *got to* make these cookies. It's a wonderful tradition in my family. It's one of the few traditions that my mother established when I was growing up. We all looked forward to it. It's a neat project for families. The kids create their own decorations. It's creative and important. We make many batches, dozens and dozens of cookies. Then we mail them out and give them out as presents."

Gail certainly was committed to those cookies—to lots and lots of those cookies! Unfortunately, cookies are committed to fat cells and increasing hunger (especially if two hundred or so are sitting around "smiling" enticingly).

Gail, her group, and I talked about this dilemma. There was no simple solution. I emphasized the biology of weight control. The group talked about using alternative artsy projects for kids. They encouraged Gail to start a new, lower-calorie tradition; they talked about spreading "the word" to friends and relatives about sugar. But how can your words encourage people to reduce consumption of sugar (and fat) when your deeds (giving the cookies) say the opposite?

Gail reacted emotionally to the idea of giving up her cookie tradition. She couldn't get herself to do it, she claimed. But she did decrease the amount of cookies she and her children baked and gave away. She also wound up munching on "too many cookies."

The next year Gail vacillated between the Frustration and Acceptance stages. She baked very few cookies during her third year in the program (but still munched on too many). Finally, the cookie tradition was replaced with the computer-generated "artistic greeting card tradition."

Gail has now lost most of the fifty pounds that she had gained over the years. She still vacillates between Frustration and Acceptance, but she spends far more time in Acceptance these days. She still munches on "too many cookies" sometimes, but avoids placing herself directly in harm's way by refusing to bake dozens of cookies for Christmas. Her weight fluctuates more than she would like. But she persists.

Step 3: Eat to Lose ▍ 105

Protein Power

"Protein" comes from the Greek word *proteios,* which means "of prime importance." According to Dr. T. Colin Campbell, nutritionist at Cornell University and author of an amazing book about nutrition and health, *The China Study* (BenBella Books, 2005), "Ever since the discovery of this nitrogen-containing chemical in 1839 by the Dutch chemist Gerhard Mulder, protein has loomed as the most sacred of all nutrients. It is still touted as the most important building block of life by most people today."

We only need about fifty grams of protein per day, but many current diets recommend consuming more than twice that amount. Current dietary recommendations (from the Institute of Medicine) include a level of protein intake ranging from about 40 to 120 grams per day. These numbers are based on the current Dietary Reference Intakes (DRIs). That range varies tremendously based on such factors as activity levels and amounts of muscle being maintained. If we consume about 10% of our total calories from protein, then virtually all of us will supply our bodies with adequate amounts of protein. In the United States, we consume 50% more than that level on average. For many weight controllers who are actively attempting to lose weight, 10% of calories from a total intake of 1,200 to 1,500 calories per day would equal only thirty to forty grams of protein per day.

In our Wellspring programs, we target seventy grams of protein per day. This level, about twice the minimal number of protein grams required for nutritional health, has been associated, at least in our experience, with substantial weight loss without much hunger or many complaints about the food. You may wish to aim for seventy grams of protein a day as a starting point to see how this affects your appetite control and your pattern of weight loss.

Protein can help you control your weight in several ways. These include:

- Stimulating the release of the digestive hormone known as CCK.
- Increased release of neurotransmitters associated with feelings of satiety and fullness. CCK helps trigger this release.
- Stabilizing your blood glucose levels by slowing digestion. The brain monitors these blood glucose levels to affect appetite when they get too low.
- Releasing of neurotransmitters in the brain that decrease hunger.

A recent review by Dr. R. J. Stubbs from The Rowett Research Institute in England (*International Journal of Obesity*, 1995) of the effects of protein versus carbohydrates versus fat on appetite led to the following conclusion:

> The data derived from a number of sources ranging from diet surveys to whole body calorimetry and nutrient infusion studies suggest that in the short-to-medium term, protein is more satiating than carbohydrate, which is more satiating than fat.

One simple way of thinking about these findings concerns the complexity of protein molecules. Protein molecules are far more complex than carbohydrate or fat molecules. This complexity causes the body to take more time to digest high-protein foods, resulting in a time-release effect on the amount of glucose (sugar) in our bloodstreams. The specific qualities of protein also trigger the release of chemicals in the brain (neurotransmitters) somewhat similar to Prozac and other antidepressants. To obtain these effects consistently, it helps to eat protein consistently throughout the day.

Protein exists in a great many foods, but especially rich sources of protein include legumes (seed-bearing plants like soybeans, green beans, peas, lentils, and kidney beans), egg whites, and lean meats (fish, seafood, and the white meats of poultry). For example, a half-cup of legumes and one ounce of lean meat each contain about ten grams of protein.

A CAVEAT ABOUT ANIMAL VERSUS PLANT PROTEIN: PLANT PROTEIN IS PROBABLY BETTER FOR YOUR HEALTH

In a very important series of studies, *The China Study's* Dr. Campbell and his associates showed that relatively high levels of animal proteins can increase the development of cancerous cells and tumors in mice and rats which have similar protein needs to humans. Dr. Campbell used strains of rats and mice that were exposed to a high level of carcinogens (chemicals that reliably produce cancerous tumors over time). He found that providing these animals with diets containing 20% of their calories from animal protein caused dramatic increases in both precancerous cells (called "foci") and actual lethal tumors over time. Quite remarkably, diets containing 5% animal protein and 20% plant protein did not produce these very harmful effects. Chart 4.2 shows these effects in a study that compared the effects of casein

CHART 4.2: PROTEIN TYPE AND FOCI RESPONSE

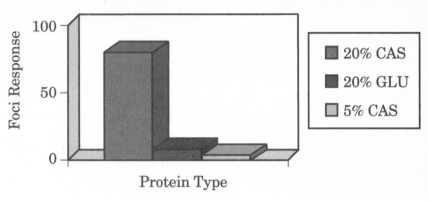

The development of precancerous cells (Foci) in rats is greatly increased by a fairly high level (20% of calories consumed per day) of animal protein ("casein"—a milk protein) but not by vegetable protein ("gluten"—a protein derived from wheat) or by a low level of animal protein (5%). Based on a study by Dr. Colin Campbell and his associates, summarized in *The China Study* by Colin Campbell (BenBella Books, 2005, p. 60, reprinted with permission).

(cow's milk protein) with gluten (wheat protein) on precancerous cell formations (foci).

Related findings have apparently been obtained for other types of proteins and other types of cancers based on studies by Dr. Campbell's group and other researchers. However, in *The China Study* (which summarizes these and other related findings), Dr. Campbell provided the following caution when applying these studies to our lives:

> So much consistency [in the animal studies] was stunningly impressive, but one aspect of this research demanded that we remain cautious: all this evidence was gathered in experimental animal studies. Although there are strong arguments that these provocative findings are *qualitatively* relevant to human health, we cannot know the *quantitative* relevance. In other words, are these principles regarding animal protein and cancer critically important for all humans in all situations, or are they merely marginally important for a minority of people in fairly unique situations (p. 66).

Dr. Campbell and his associates ventured far outside their laboratories in Ithaca, New York, to see if their impressive findings about the potential dangers of animal protein might emerge in humans. They conducted a massive nutritional study in China that involved almost one billion people over twenty years. This study also showed that a diet very low in fat, high in fiber, and low in animal protein seems clearly associated with very low incidences of heart disease, cancer, and other serious afflictions in affluent cultures like ours. However, even the least active groups of Chinese people who were studied are more active than the vast majority of Americans. So, increased activity was also associated with improved health, as we would expect.

The China Study's results were consistent with the animal studies, but such survey research doesn't prove that animal protein at modest levels with an approach like the Wellspring Plan will prove harmful for most people, most of the time. The Wellspring Plan encourages a very low-fat and high-fiber diet, as well as greatly increased activity levels. Further research may show that even in this context, much smaller amounts of animal protein than expected can produce harmful results. The most cautious approach would be to attempt to eliminate as much animal protein (and fat) from your diet as possible. A less stringent approach would be to aim for no more than forty grams of animal protein per day, which would be less than 10% of calories from protein for most weight controllers. The latter level would provide some protection, as shown by another one of Dr. Campbell's findings (Chart 4.3). Note that precancerous foci didn't develop at an accelerated level until a 12% animal protein diet was consumed by the rats in this study.

Following even the least restrictive recommendation (forty grams of animal protein per day) will prove quite challenging to many people. You will find yourself consuming more soy milk, low-fat tofu, Seitan (a wheat protein meat substitute), and legumes in order to satisfy your appetite and maximize your long-term health. Fortunately, these foods are becoming more widely available in very convenient forms, including frozen low-fat soy cheese pizzas and many other products. Sources of animal protein are among the more calorie-dense foods people in the Wellspring Plan typically consume. This approach will, therefore, also encourage eating foods that are low in calories and in energy density, an important element of the Wellspring Plan, as described in the next section of this chapter. Many of the recipes featured in Chapter 11 feature vegetarian dishes that are enjoyable and easy to make, which will help you lower your intake of animal protein.

CHART 4.3: FOCI PROMOTION BY DIETARY PROTEIN

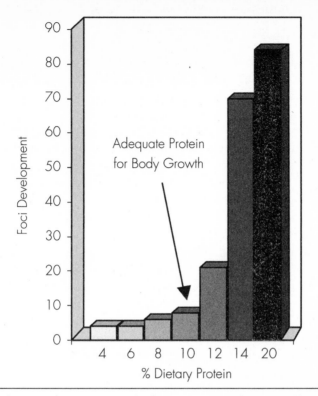

The development of precancerous cells (foci) in rats is greatly increased by relatively high levels of consumption of animal protein, but not by lower levels. Based on studies published by Dr. Colin Campbell and his associates, summarized in *The China Study* by Colin Campbell (BenBella Books, 2005, p.57, reprinted with permission).

Soup City: Low Energy Density

If you could eat as much as you wanted in order to feel satisfied, in which of the following meals would you wind up consuming more total calories?

Grilled chicken, seasoned white rice, assorted vegetables, and a glass of ice water	Soup made from grilled chicken, seasoned white rice, assorted vegetables, and water

Several studies suggest it would take about 20% more of the non-soup meal to make you feel full, in part because you would not consume as much water during the meal, giving it a higher energy density. The soup, on the other hand, has fewer calories per gram because of the amount of liquid in it. Its high water content both gives it a lower energy density and causes you to feel fuller more quickly. In everyday life, foods that are low in energy density include vegetables, fruits, and very low-fat foods. Foods with the highest energy density would be such things as chocolate, pastries, and high-fat meats and cheeses.

Quite a few studies have shown that people eat considerably less of meals containing more fluid (low energy density) than they do with the same fat levels in higher-density presentations. Some of these studies also show that simply removing some high-density foods from a person's diet has little effect on their total consumption. On the other hand, removing all sources of high-fat foods almost always results in much less eating in general and a much lower fat intake.

Eating low-density foods increases the size of the stomach, which creates a feeling of fullness. Eating such foods also slows down the rate of transfer of nutrients into the small intestines, another mechanism that decreases appetite and increases feelings of fullness.

A study of nearly 1,800 participants conducted in Philadelphia nicely illustrates this point. Greater consumption of soup was associated with better weight loss. Perhaps similar findings would occur if the researchers measured consumptions of salads per week or eating large portions of vegetables every day.

The take-away message from research on energy density is that you will find weight control easier if you focus on low-density foods. In particular, try to eat as much low-fat soup as you can and order lots of vegetables when dining out. This will make you feel more satisfied more often, as well as decrease your desire to eat higher-fat foods.

Roughing It: Fiber

Health writer Ruth Papazian recently argued that fiber was the Rodney Dangerfield of food: it got no respect. Fiber, sometimes called roughage, can cause gas, bloating, and other unpleasant side effects (think baked beans). These occasional unpleasant moments deserve the Dangerfield treatment far more than fiber. Fiber can decrease appetite, improve weight loss, and reduce the risk of heart disease and some cancers. How is that for respectable?

Definition. According to the Food and Drug Administration and the Institute of Medicine (a non-governmental group of experts hired to write scientific reports for the public), fiber is a nutrient composed of non-digestible carbohydrates. More specifically:

- Dietary fiber consists of non-digestible carbohydrates that are intrinsic and intact in plants.
- Added fiber consists of isolated, non-digestible carbohydrates which have beneficial physiological effects in humans.
- Total fiber is the sum of dietary and added fiber.

FIBER AND WEIGHT

Populations that consume lots of fiber have relatively few overweight people. In Kenya, Uganda, and Malawi, for example, where less than 15% of adults are overweight, people eat more than four times the fiber we do (sixty to eight grams per day versus fifteen grams per day). Could it be mere coincidence that we eat one-quarter the fiber but have four times the percentage of overweight people of these high-fiber countries? Here's another statistic worth pondering: even within each country, those who consume more fiber weigh less than those who consume very little fiber.

An important study published by Drs. Alfieri, Pomerleau, Grace, and Anderson (*Obesity Research*, 1995) compared the effects of providing a fiber supplement versus a placebo supplement to overweight participants. The participants who got the fiber lost significantly more weight and reported significantly less hunger than the placebo group. Fiber supplementation has also improved the maintenance of weight loss in other research.

HOW FIBER HELPS

Fiber acts to reduce the energy density of foods consumed. Adding large quantities of high-fiber vegetables to a meal increases the bulk and weight of the food while barely influencing the amount of calories consumed. Consider the example of adding lettuce, tomatoes, and bean sprouts to a sandwich and changing the bread from white to whole grain. These veggies might add thirty calories and the change in bread would add no additional calories, but those changes would add about six grams of fiber (20% of the day's goal for fiber).

High-fiber foods also increase chewing, promoting increased production of saliva and stomach acids. Those fluids and the bulk of the food can increase distention of the stomach and decrease the speed of absorption in the intestines. These effects increase feelings of satiation (satisfaction of appetite during eating) and satiety (fullness): satiation + satiety = decreased eating.

RECOMMENDATION: A MINIMUM OF THIRTY GRAMS OF FIBER PER DAY

Health and nutrition experts (for example, those at the Institute of Medicine) recommend that we double our current intake of fiber from fifteen grams to thirty grams per day. As a weight controller, you need all the help you can get to fight your resistant biology and the excess hunger this unfortunate biology awakens in you every day. Eating plenty of fiber, in addition to soups, can lower your diet's energy density and increase your satisfaction. So, consider using some of the following foods regularly to get to a minimum of thirty grams of fiber every day:

- High-fiber breakfast cereals, such as Raisin Bran (1 cup = 8 grams), Multi-Bran Chex (1 cup = 8 grams), and bulgur (cracked wheat, 1 cup = 8 grams)
- Whole grain breads for sandwiches (2 slices = 4 grams)
- Bean soups or ¼ cup of baked beans or ½ cup of peas, lentils, or corn (all = 5 grams)
- 1 medium-sized white potato with skin or 1 cup of brown rice or ½ cup of whole grain pasta (all = 4 grams)
- 3 to 4 servings of veggies or salad (1/2 cup = 6 grams)
- fresh fruit (1 medium-sized fruit = 1 serving = 3 grams)

In addition to these suggestions consider some side-by-side comparisons and decide which would work best for you:

- White bread (1 slice): 75 calories, 1g fat, 0.7g fiber versus whole grain bread: 2g fiber (same calories and fat)
- White rice (1 cup cooked): 240 cal, 0.5g fat, 1.6g fiber versus brown rice (1 cup cooked): 220 calories, 1.5g fat, 3.2g fiber
- Orange juice (1 12-ounce glass): 165 calories, 0g fat, 0.5g fiber versus oranges (2 medium-sized): 140 calories, 0g fat, 7.6g fiber

The first two side-by-side comparisons suggest the strong benefit of adding color to your grain selections whenever possible. This even works for potatoes, with sweetpotatoes having 50% more fiber than white potatoes. The last comparison indicates that as famed nutritionist Allan

Borushek, the "Calorie King" (see www.calorieking.com), pointed out, when you eat fresh fruit instead of the juice, you consume more fiber and fewer calories, spend considerable time chewing, and have better satisfaction (reduced hunger), slower absorption, and less release of insulin. Now, *that* is a nutritional deal few weight controllers can pass up!

CONCLUSION ABOUT FIBER: IMPLICATIONS FOR THE WELLSPRING PLAN

As someone striving to develop your *Wellspring Plan*, you might appreciate the importance of the emphasis on setting a daily goal for fiber. Healthy obsessions require routines—powerful ones that remind you of your program and its importance. To reach a minimum intake goal of thirty or more grams of fiber every day, you'll find yourself ordering double portions of vegetables at restaurants, munching carrots regularly, insisting on whole grain bread for your sandwiches, seeking out whole fruits for snacks, and making or ordering soups very often. Those routines will reinforce your focus on activity, very low-fat foods, and consistent self-monitoring. The more you embrace these routines and make them truly significant parts of your lives, the stronger your *Wellspring Plan*—and the better your chances for lifelong success.

Minimal Liquid Calories: Eat Your Calories—Don't Drink Them

In the previous section, you read about the substantial benefits of eating fresh oranges versus drinking orange juice. The following recent research findings show the problems caused by drinking any calorie-laden sweet drinks (including sodas, sports drinks, and fruit juices):

- Researchers from Denmark provided overweight volunteers with either sugared soda or diet sodas. The volunteers ate freely otherwise over the ten-week study. Those who drank sugared sodas consumed an extra five hundred to seven hundred calories a day and gained an average of three-and-one-half pounds. They also increased their blood pressures. Those who drank diet sodas lost two pounds.
- In a study conducted at Purdue University, volunteers were assessed during a baseline period to determine how many calories they typically consumed. Then, during two four-week experimental periods, they were given 18% of their baseline calories as either jelly beans (solid sugar calories) or sugared soda (liquid

calories). When the volunteers ate the jelly beans, they compensated for the calories in the jelly beans by eating less during the day. In this way, the jelly beans had no effect on their total consumption of calories or weight compared to their baselines. In contrast, when they consumed the sugared sodas, they ate more total calories and gained weight.

- Dr. David Ludwig and his associates at Harvard University found that for each additional sugared drink (such as juice, soda, or a sports drink) consumed by middle-school children, compared to the average middle-schooler, there was a 60% increased risk for the development of obesity—even after controlling for the influence of lifestyle and diet.

Even though sugared drinks contain no fat, they clearly create problems for weight controllers. Even the American Pediatric Association now recommends diet sodas over fruit juices for this reason. Fruit juice—even 100% fruit juice—provides almost no fiber and lots of concentrated sugary calories—calories that apparently increase total calories consumed per day.

The major exception to this dictum (eat your calories—don't drink them) involves skim milk. Skim milk contains good amounts of protein (nine grams per glass) and lots of calcium. Some research even shows that consuming lots of dairy products and calcium (in addition to protein) may help you lose weight. So, the bottom line is: Eat your calories—don't drink them (except for skim milk).

Drinking occasional light beer and wine also won't destroy your weight control program. These drinks may be important to you in order for you to find foods (and some drinks) you love that love you back (see the next chapter for more on this key point). On the other hand, if you drink alcohol frequently or excessively on occasion, that could certainly affect your *Wellspring Plan*. A healthy obsession depends on your ability to stay focused. An alcohol-induced high can cause your focus to drift, and suddenly chips, nuts, and fried chicken wings seem perfectly okay. Also, alcoholic drinks contain plenty of calories, especially the colorful kinds that come with small paper umbrellas in them.

Calorie Consciousness

If you ate unlimited quantities of very low-fat, high-plant protein, low-density, low-sugar, high-fiber foods, then you would certainly gain a substantial amount of weight. These five elements of eating to lose weight can control your appetite and regulate your weight; however, you have to watch what happens on the scale as you implement the *Wellspring Plan.* If your activity levels have increased substantially and you are following these food guidelines but your weight doesn't change, then you have to consider focusing more specifically on the amount of calories you are consuming every day.

The highly successful weight controllers in the National Weight Control Registry studies have lost more than fifty pounds and maintain that weight loss for an average of six years. Their reported average intake per day is approximately 1,350 calories. Based on prior research that verifies reports of eating, it seems likely that this number is a bit low. Let's assume their average intake is closer to 1,500 or 1,600 calories per day as a maintenance level. These numbers suggest that a good target for weight loss for most people might be 1,200 to 1,300 calories per day, in addition to considerable activity. If you are able to lose weight consistently simply by following the other six elements in this chapter and increasing your activity levels, then you needn't focus very specifically on the calories consumed. However, to accelerate weight loss or to begin weight loss for some people, these levels of caloric consumption can guide your eating. In addition, many of my clients find that one other caloric guideline has proven particularly helpful:

Consume no more than eight hundred calories
at your biggest meal of the day.

A 2004 report from the Centers for Disease Control shows why attention to calorie consumption matters. According to this report, men now eat 168 more calories daily than they did in 1971. They now eat, according to self-reports, approximately 2,600 calories a day. Women now consume 335 more calories, increasing their total calorie consumption to approximately 1,900 calories per day. Most nutritionists would argue that these self-reports are probably lower than reality. For example, Dr. Susan Roberts of the Energy Metabolism Lab at Tufts University noted, "We're now at the point that more than six in ten Americans are either overweight or obese. We didn't get there on 1,900 to 2,600 calories per day. U.S. food supply data indicate we're eating considerably more."

This means that if you are a serious weight controller, you'll consume about half of what the average American consumes per day. You'll also expend far more energy than typical Americans and eat more fiber and more low-density food. The dramatic differences between you and the average American demonstrates one reason why a healthy obsession is so critical to success at long-term weight control. When you deviate so much from the average tendencies of those around you, you must rely on a good deal of inner strength to stay the course.

Exceptions?

The *Wellspring Plan* takes a strong position against moderation as a useful approach to long-term success. Most health professionals don't agree with this and advise their clients that it is just fine to have high-fat foods some of the time. These professionals, however well-intentioned, are usually not experts on, or if they have some expertise in this arena, do not understand the science behind the *Wellspring Plan*. In the *Wellspring Plan* every instance of high-fat eating is considered a problem, not a disaster, but certainly a problem. Let's consider some responses to common questions about this unusual, but critical, aspect of the *Wellspring Plan*.

QUESTION: *What about having pizza at least every once in a while? Pizza, after all, has all of the food groups.*
ANSWER: Pizzas often contain vegetables, dairy, meat, and grains; they do, indeed, provide a wide range of food groups. However, pizza also contains a good number of calories, many of which come from fat. For example, two slices of a national fast food pizza chain's stuffed pizza contains 860 calories and forty grams of fat (42% of the calories come from fat). Even this pizza chain's less caloric pizzas, as well as the largest national chain's full range of pizza offerings, contain 30 to 40% of their calories from fat. That's three to four times more than your goal in the *Wellspring Plan*!

The good news is that many places will serve pizzas without any cheese, which does represent a good food choice. The crust in most pizzas contains some fat (usually one to two grams per slice), but as an alternative food, pizzas with no cheese can work very well.

If you are trapped in a party or meeting and surrounded by pizzas, what can you do? You can perform minor surgery and remove the cheese from your pizza. Some people may find this distasteful and although it may not be the most acceptable form of behavior, it could work much better for you than eating high-fat food and compromising your *Wellspring Plan*.

QUESTION: *What about frozen yogurt?*
ANSWER: Most frozen yogurts are enjoyable low-fat desserts. However, some of them can be surprisingly high in fat content and, therefore, deviate from the plan. If you are selective and read labels carefully, you can find very low-fat or no-fat frozen yogurts or sorbets. But remember, most frozen yogurts contain lots of sugar or other sweeteners that could trigger some of the same reactions other sugary foods do.

Many weight controllers use frozen yogurt in modest amounts as a treat, which is a good approach. Just be careful of some establishments that serve nearly twice the amounts they advertise for a given price. Try ordering the smallest, child-size portion available at a frozen yogurt stand or restaurant or purchase frozen yogurt or sorbet popsicles. Frozen yogurt can also become problematic if it is purchased in pints, quarts, or larger bulk quantities. Many people find themselves dipping into these treats more often than desirable. So the answer is: use frozen yogurt with caution.

QUESTION: *What about birthday cake (traditional high-fat type with icing)?*
ANSWER: Birthday cakes are an important tradition to many people. However, traditions can change. Why would you want to eat a food that creates a problem for you in celebration of a special day? When you first had a birthday cake to celebrate your birthday during childhood, you didn't realize the kind of problem foods high in sugar and fat create for you. In fact, at that time, you probably didn't have such a problem. Now, you have new information that advises against consuming foods like cake. In the 1950s, practically every dinner table in America had red meat on it, but that tradition has changed. It is now time for you to consider changing the birthday cake tradition for yourself. This position may seem rather extreme, but weight control takes extreme focusing and persistence. If you really want to succeed at this difficult challenge, you must take difficult steps.

Another problem with allowing yourself birthday cake is that if you give yourself permission for this deviation from the plan, what else will you permit? What about other holidays? What about other people's birthdays? What about your children's birthdays? Some of the clients with whom I have worked give themselves permission to eat problematic foods when they are hungry, tired, on vacation, at someone else's house for dinner or for a party, or when they are sad or depressed. The list goes on and on. Permissions often create problems. For example, if you give yourself permission to eat problematic food today, then you may struggle mightily with other food decisions tomorrow. These struggles take their toll. Instead of food becoming more secondary in your life, the struggle becomes primary. Lots of struggles can put you into a major Frustration stage—an unpleasant stage that often produces unfavorable results. Can all of these problems come from a birthday cake? Perhaps!

QUESTION: *How can you tell about sauces in restaurants?*
ANSWER: You can assume that any sauce made in a restaurant with oil as a primary ingredient is problematic. On the other hand, tomato sauces and sauces that are essentially broths (which are available increasingly in restaurants) are quite acceptable. Any sauces made with cheese (such as Alfredo sauce) are very high in fat; similarly, sauces and soups with cream bases are very high-fat foods. One of my clients recently told a story about a seemingly innocuous mushroom soup which her dining companion ordered. Her companion raved about how wonderful the soup was, and it looked very appealing to the client. But when she tasted the soup, she soon realized that its primary ingredient was butter. The word "mushroom" suggests a low-fat, safe, vegetable base. As Americans become increasingly health-conscious, restaurateurs and food packagers will market and name products to suggest their healthfulness. You can generally assume that if you're not sure about the ingredients in a product, it's best to avoid it, and if you do know the ingredients, avoid those high in fat and sugar. These guidelines may sound stringent, but unfortunately your biology demands such stringencies. Successful weight controllers follow these guidelines with tremendous consistency.

Eating and Cancer:
Can You Prevent Cancer by Eating Better?

Cancer strikes ten million people a year. Three to four million of those cases could have been prevented through healthier eating and exercising. In fact, eating more fruits and vegetables alone could eliminate as many as two million new cases of cancer a year.

In 1997, the World Cancer Research Fund and the American Institute for Cancer Research issued a comprehensive report on the relationship between eating and cancer. This report, based on a careful review of more than 4,500 studies, stressed that no food or drink can prevent cancer, but concluded that a diet that emphasizes certain foods can certainly lower your risk of getting this deadly disease.

In addition to decreasing consumption of animal protein based on the research described in *The China Study*, five eating and drinking strategies that almost certainly can decrease the risk of getting cancer are:

1. **Eat lots of vegetables.** The average American eats only three or four servings a day of vegetables. Five servings are clearly preferable and nine are recommended by virtually all nutritional experts. Yellow, dark green, and orange vegetables rich in carotenoids and all the cabbage family vegetables (broccoli, brussels sprouts, cauliflower, collards, kale, bok choy, and mustard/turnip greens) all seem to lower the risk of cancer. Garlic, onions, and leeks may also help ward off cancer, especially breast cancer.

2. **Eat lots of fruits.** Fruits rich in Vitamin C (all citrus fruits, tomatoes, and strawberries) are especially helpful. Fruits are great examples of low-density foods and can be enjoyed several times a day without creating problems for most weight controllers.

3. **Decrease consumption of total fat—particularly saturated fat.** This panel recommended that fats provide between 15 and 30% of total calories. You may recall that I have recommended that you go "as low as you can go" in total fat—for most this may amount to 5 to 10% of your total calories from fat.

4. **Decrease alcohol consumption; limit drinks to fewer than two a day for men and one a day for women.** The panel concluded that although alcohol may have some benefits for decreasing heart disease when consumed in small amounts, the risk for cancers—particularly breast, colon, and rectal cancers—is significant. People who consume even small amounts of alcohol have a significantly greater chance of developing cancer than those who do not drink alcohol at all.

5. **The following foods and drinks may also help reduce the risk of cancer, at least somewhat: dried beans, milk, fish, green tea, whole grain cereals, and olive oil.** The evidence favoring these particular foods and drinks is not as convincing as the evidence in the first four recommendations. Nonetheless, the panel concluded those items may prove beneficial and are worth including in healthy eating plans.

Summary and Conclusions

The Seven Elements of Eating to Lose are reprinted below to help summarize the seven key principles of eating and drinking in the *Wellspring Plan*. Focusing on consuming as little fat as possible will help you implement the other six elements. When you eat a very low-fat diet, you will naturally gravitate to low-density foods because fat is by far the most calorically dense nutrient (nine calories per gram versus four calories per gram for protein and carbs). Decreasing fat also leads to eating few animal sources of protein. For example, the vast majority of red meats are very high in fat. Low-density and low-fat foods also have lots of fiber, and so on. So, start your focus with the goal of near-zero fat intake and you'll get to the most healthful diet, full of foods you love that love you back.

SEVEN ELEMENTS OF EATING TO LOSE

1. **Fat**: Eat very little fat (aim for zero fat grams per day, accept up to twenty grams per day). Importance =1
2. **Sugar**: Minimize sugar when snacking. Avoid sugary foods (like candy bars or lollipops) as stand-alone snacks. Importance = 6
3. **Protein**: Eat lean sources of protein frequently throughout the day, substituting plant for animal sources as much as possible (seventy grams of total protein per day; fewer than forty grams of this from animal protein). Importance = 6
4. **Low-Density Foods**: Eat/drink lots of low-fat soups and other foods that are low in "energy density." Importance = 2
5. **Fiber**: Eat at least thirty grams of fiber (non-digestible parts of plant foods) per day. Importance = 7
6. **Drinks**: Eat your calories—don't drink them. Importance = 4
7. **Calories**: Maintain calorie consciousness (goal for maximum calories at you're your biggest meal of the day = 800). Importance = 2

Epilogue: Does Eating Right Cost Too Much?

Do you think that buying fresh fruits and vegetables, even in the dead of winter, will break your bank account? Researchers have found that four out of ten people believe that buying fruits, vegetables, fish, and other healthful foods, particularly out of season, costs more than the items they currently buy. But this is just not true.

When researchers gave several hundred people with high cholesterol levels videos that showed them how to cut fat from their diets, those whose cholesterol levels dropped the most after nine months decreased their food bills by more than a dollar a day.

Consider the cost differences between a doughnut or a muffin bought at a convenience store and cereal with skim milk. The cereal and skim milk will cost quite a bit less than the surprisingly pricey bakery goods. Consider another example: Do you think twice about spending three dollars on a pint of your favorite pseudo-import frozen yogurt? What about spending the same three dollars for a pint of strawberries in the dead of winter to top that frozen yogurt? You may resist spending money for the strawberries, but not for the frozen yogurt. Compare the three dollars spent on the pint of frozen yogurt or on a grande latte versus three dollars for six frozen veggie burgers.

Even if your appetite tends toward rather pricey fruits and vegetables in the off-season, consider how much time and energy and money you put into the effort to stay healthy and lose weight. You can follow the seven elements economically or spend a bit more for off-season fruits and vegetables. After all, isn't that asparagus worth it? Aren't you worth it?

Step 4: Find Lovable Foods that Love You Back

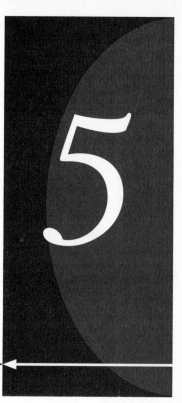

"THE THING I LOVE ABOUT A GOOD STEAK is its hardiness; its stick-to-your-ribs quality. It just looks and smells like it's going to feel so good going down. I like it burned around the edges, pinkish in the middle, sizzling hot. I know I'll feel satisfied and nicely full and relaxed after a good steak. Steaks may cost some serious bucks, but they're a lot cheaper than Prozac."

"A couple of scoops of really rich chocolate or vanilla fudge ice cream just call out to me sometimes. I just love the smooth creamy texture and the taste sensation of rich ice cream. It creates this 'ahh' and 'yum' feeling that is simultaneously exciting and relaxing. What else in life does that? Well, I guess I can think of something—but you can't buy *that* twenty-four hours a day at your nearest convenience store. Or maybe you can but I just don't know how."

"Nothing smells as good as freshly baked chocolate chip cookies! I mean nothing. When they just come out of the oven, piping hot, they really take over the room. They bring me back to a simpler time, with my brother and sister happily laughing and excitedly arguing about who gets the first one. That melt-in-your-mouth warmth and sweetness is just one of the great parts of being human."

What makes your favorite foods lovable? According to my clients, lovable foods have certain qualities in common:

- Look really good
- Taste great
- Have mouth appeal—chewy or crunchy or just right for the moment
- Smell great
- Create good, happy, and satisfied feelings
- Are craved for their special qualities
- Have nostalgic value, reminders of something good from the past, like warm family gatherings or very relaxing or romantic moments
- Provide comfort and relief from stress

Such qualities abound in juicy steaks, rich ice creams, and freshly baked cookies. I have heard friends describe, in amazing detail, the lovable qualities of freshly baked lemon meringue pies, rich beers, and perfect pizzas. We talk about such foods with a certain reverence, elevating them to romantic heights.

Weight controllers need this passion for food. Living the good life includes enjoying good food, and if you aren't passionate about your food and thus minimize your interest in it, making food bland and unappealing, you can expect to fail in the quest for permanent change. Among the thousands of clients I have worked with over the past thirty years, those who have achieved long-term success have kept the passion in their food and in other parts of their lives. In short, by cherishing your passion for food, you can help yourself lose weight permanently.

Four Aspects of Lovable Foods

If you learn the details about the lovability of food, you might be able to increase your enjoyment of it and your passion for it. Identifying these qualities is just the beginning of understanding how passion for food really works. Consider your reaction if you went to a fancy, expensive restaurant and all the food was presented wrapped in layers of paper, like a fast-food meal. Would that presentation affect your reaction to the food? What if you ordered chicken soup on a cold wintry day and it came out cold and clammy? Would a frozen yogurt cone appeal to you as much if it were served warm and drippy?

Obviously, lovability in foods goes far beyond mere taste sensations. Restaurants go to great pains to set the stage for their food. They know that presentation affects lovability in their foods and they want you to love their food—and come back for more, again and again. To assist you in your quest to find lovable foods that love you back, let's consider all the factors that affect the appeal of food. By increasing your awareness of each factor, you can get more lovability out of your food.

The following are four aspects of food that affect their appeal or lovability:

Taste
- sweet
- salty
- sour
- bitter

Appearance
- attractive, beautiful
- unattractive, ugly
- pleasing setting
- fresh
- stale, spoiled

Smell
- pleasing, appropriate for type of food
- displeasing, foul, inappropriate
- strong versus weak

Texture
- creamy
- crunchy
- chalky
- smooth
- chewy

Taste, the most obvious one, consists of various combinations of sweet, sour, salty, and bitter. Consider the simple pretzel, for example. If you eat a pretzel in a quiet, dark room—and eat it slowly and attentively—you'll certainly notice the saltiness, but you'll also detect sweetness. You might even find that the inside of the pretzel, the dry white stuff, tastes a little bitter, at least compared to the outside's salty-sweet shell.

What happens if you pay attention to each aspect of taste? My clients say that they appreciate and enjoy their food more when they get themselves to do this. Pretzels, formerly a quick salty snack, become something that is a little sweet, quite salty, a little bitter, and a lot more interesting and enjoyable.

Now what happens if you put the pretzels on a hand-crafted oak platter, next to several porcelain cups with various mustards in them, on top of a glistening round antique oak table? Wouldn't their appeal increase compared to the appeal of pretzels being eaten right out of the bag in your car? Appearance definitely matters. Smell and texture in food also matter. If your pretzels were stale, rubbery, or smelled funny, you'd find them less lovable. If you like coffee, you know that a strong coffee smell, an appealing mug, and a cozy setting in which to drink it all affect its lovability.

You can use all four aspects of the lovability of food to make your low-fat world much more enjoyable. Consider trying the following lovability enhancers as often as possible:

- Accentuate taste by eating slowly and attempting to identify the degree to which whatever you eat tastes sweet, salty, sour, and/ or bitter. You can think of this as savoring your food by making yourself aware of each element of its taste.
- Maximize the appearance of food that you serve yourself. This applies even when eating your food out of a microwavable box. It helps to put the food on a nice plate and sit down at a pleasant table for your meal. You can try adding candles, place settings, and flowers to create your own beautiful ambiance.
- Enjoy smells of food. All food smells are both fat-free and calorie-free! You can try this at coffee shops, cheese counters, and other places where strong appealing smells waft through the air. For your own food, take time to identify the smells and notice what you enjoy about each of them.
- Pay attention to texture in everything you eat. You can enjoy

luxurious textures in very low-fat foods quite readily. Can you think of chewy fat-free foods that you sometimes enjoy? (Hint: gum, turkey jerky.) Certainly frozen yogurts can vary in creaminess, and lots of healthful snacks have plenty of crunch, like carrots, pretzels, and most fresh vegetables. For smooth qualities, smoothies and even certain cereals can prove satisfying.

Sweetpotatoes: a Lovable Food that Loves You Back

Lovable foods can certainly, definitely, and without a doubt include foods that *love you back*. Foods that help you lose weight, achieve your goals, make you healthier, and are constructive rather than destructive can fulfill all of the qualities of traditional lovable foods.

The same clients who waxed poetic about steaks and chocolate sundaes have talked lovingly about sweetpotatoes:

- "Sweetpotatoes are treats: colorful, easy, tasty."
- "They fill me up—and do it with warmth and flavor."
- "They remind me of holidays—obviously Thanksgiving, but also Christmas. I remember the sweet smell of them, bubbling out of the oven with marshmallows on top. Definite yums for yams from my family."
- "They're interesting; you can do so much with them—make them crunchy or soupy or top them with a whole world of possibilities. Usually I top them with honey mustard for a sweet and tangy taste, but they also work really well with different fruit salsas or barbecue sauces or yogurts."
- "I know that when I get home I'm nine minutes away from something sweet, filling, and satisfying."

My clients talk about remembering Thanksgiving and the comfort and warmth of family. Certainly not all of their families were warm and comfortable, nor was Thanksgiving always a wonderful, satisfying experience. Yet positive memories for most of us include the smells of turkey and sweetpotatoes filling the house on a cold, brisk afternoon, intermingling with a crackling wood fire and the sounds of a football game echoing from a nearby television.

Sweetpotatoes have their place as a warm, comfortable, celebratory food in many of our hearts and minds. Can you see a sweetpotato casserole in your memory and remember the "oohs" and "aahs" from the family gathered together? Can you remember the feeling of warm excitement that you felt as a child when the food first came out of the oven? Lovable foods can bring these associations back to life.

As with all lovable foods, you can eat sweetpotatoes with gusto. One of my clients, Casey, said she could keep losing weight "as long as the sweetpotato farmers stay in business." She likes their convenience, warmth, taste, amazing filling quality, variations (with different toppings, for example), and smell. Casey's story, below, highlights her sheer enjoyment of food, eaten now as a successful weight controller:

Casey: A Sweetpotato a Day

Casey described her struggle with weight control as something that was always with her. She was preoccupied by "my fat, my pathetic eating." At fifty years old and five feet six inches tall, she weighed 242 pounds when she first came to my office. Many areas of her life seemed to be fine. But her eating and her weight "just seemed hopeless." Every day she felt annoyed and disappointed in herself: "My kids love and trust me. I've got this great new job, full of challenges and prospects. Barry, my love, is wonderful. How can I keep myself so miserable by eating like I do?"

The very first week she started my program she made an immediate transformation to very low-fat eating, daily exercising, extended walks both to and from her car and during the lunch hour, and careful journaling of her eating and exercising. By far the most dramatic change in her life was the discovery that she could love to eat foods that could love her back. She began having sweetpotatoes every day for dinner, really big ones that she dressed up in various ways. She was shocked by how much she could really enjoy healthy eating. Enjoyment was the key and sweetpotatoes were the most enjoyable food she rediscovered. She found ways of loving foods that were constructive, not destructive. Although her job involved going to restaurants, she learned to make every type of restaurant work for her. Over and over again, as her weight decreased by one to two pounds per week, she was surprised and pleased by how wonderful it felt to finally be getting her problem under control.

One year and fifty-seven pounds later, Casey still expresses wonder at the quality of her food and the amazing transformations in her life. She loves her new clothes and the sense of strength that she has enjoyed by increasing her exercising and her everyday activities. On many occasions she has talked about not being able to imagine ever going back to eating foods with even modest amounts of fat in them. She says, "Why should I eat other things? I really love sweetpotatoes and the rest of this stuff. If you look for it, it's all around you and it's just wonderful!" Casey has learned that weight control can work without deprivation. It requires passion for food, comfort in food, and appreciation of foods that can love you back.

A Nutritional Champ

Sweetpotatoes are assuredly a very lovable food. Their ability to love you back has also put them at the top of the list of nutritious foods. The consumer watchdog group Center for Science in the Public Interest (CSPI) has scored qualities of foods over the years by adding up their percentages of recommended values for various vitamins, minerals, cancer-fighting elements, and fiber. Sweetpotatoes scored higher than every other food. For example, in one of CSPI's surveys a medium-sized baked sweetpotato scored 184; the next highest score was eighty-three, awarded to a medium-sized baked white potato. Another survey using a different scoring system put sweetpotatoes on top again (582 points), 148 points above carrots, the second place finisher (434 points).

The following table shows the nutrients in sweetpotatoes compared with white potatoes. As you can see, both types of potatoes are very good foods. For example, both are almost fat-free, cholesterol free, and very low in salt (sodium). But the sweetpotato stands out for several of its nutritional aspects:

- Medium-sized baked sweetpotatoes have 19.3% fewer calories than medium-sized baked white potatoes.
- Medium-sized sweetpotatoes have 50% more dietary fiber, a major aid in digestion and a means of providing fullness and assisting in hunger control. If a white potato is eaten with skin, however, that can more than double its fiber content. Very few people eat sweetpotato skins (because they are too bitter).
- Medium sweetpotatoes have about ten times the Recommended Daily Allowance of vitamin A; white potatoes have no vitamin A.
- A medium-sized sweetpotato provides three times more vitamin E than a medium-sized baked white potato. Most foods that are rich in vitamin E, such as vegetable oils, nuts, and avocados also

contain lots of fat. This makes sweetpotatoes a nutritional bargain for vitamin E because they have virtually no fat.

- A medium-sized sweetpotato provides at least 10% of the recommended levels of potassium, manganese, selenium, and zinc.

TABLE 5.1 NUTRIENTS IN POTATOES	Baked Sweetpotato	Baked White Potato
Size (g)	114	156
Calories (kcal)	117	145
Carbohydrate (g)	28	34
Protein (g)	2	3
Fat (g)	0.1	0.2
Dietary Fiber (g)	3.4	2 (eaten with skin: 4.8 g fiber)
Minerals		
Calcium (mg)	32	8
Iron (mg)	0.5	0.6
Magnesium (mg)	23	39
Manganese (mg)	0.6	0.3
Phosphorus (mg)	63	78
Potassium (mg)	397	610
Sodium (mg)	11	8
Selenium (mg)	0.8	0.5
Zinc (mg)	0.3	0.5
Copper (mg)	0.2	0.3
Vitamins		
Vitamin A (IU)	24,877	0
Vitamin C (mg)	28	20
Vitamin E (mg)	0.3	0.1
Thiamin (mg)	0.1	0.2
Riboflavin (mg)	0.1	.03
Folate (mcg)	26	14
Niacin (mg)	0.7	2.2
Pantothenic acid (mg)	0.7	0.9

These excellent nutritional qualities make it clear why dietitians place sweetpotatoes near the top of virtually all of their lists of "super-foods." Just the vitamin A content of sweetpotatoes makes them truly extraordinary, as it is needed for healthy eyes, skin, mucous membranes, bone growth, tooth development, embryonic growth, and immunity mechanisms for fighting infection and disease. Vitamin A may even help the body regulate its time clock. Deficiencies in vitamin A can cause night blindness, problems with the production of tears, and heightened vulnerability to a variety of conditions leading to complete loss of vision. Although these eye diseases are rare in the well-nourished United States, up to 500,000 children a year lose their sight because of deficiencies in vitamin A, according to a recent *Consumer Reports Newsletter* (October 2001, p. 4). Perhaps most exciting in recent years has been research showing that the building blocks for vitamin A that come from plants (the carotenoid family) may prevent several kinds of cancer, including lung, stomach, larynx, esophageal, bladder, colon, rectal, and prostate cancer. Sweetpotatoes provide a remarkable amount of beta-carotene, one of the three types of carotenoids building blocks for vitamin A (alpha-carotene and beta-cryptoxanthin are the others).

History and Variety of Sweetpotatoes

When you realize the extraordinary nutritional qualities of sweetpotatoes, you can appreciate that one of Christopher Columbus' greatest unheralded discoveries may have been the sweetpotato, which he introduced to Europe in the late 1400s, using a Native American name, written in several ways: "batatas," "patate," and "potat." Europeans then referred to sweetpotatoes as "potatoes" until the white potatoes we know landed there and were also called "potato." To create a distinction, the orange-fleshed vegetable originally called "potato" in Europe was renamed "sweet potato." In recent times, botanical classifiers have begun using the name as one word, "sweetpotato," to distinguish it definitively from the white potato.

The distinction becomes more complicated when you realize that not only do sweetpotatoes differ in many ways from potatoes, but they also differ dramatically from what we call "yams." The sweetpotato is a member of the plant family known as the "morning glory," a prehistoric vegetable that serves as a root to store fluids and food for a larger plant. The most common varieties in the United States are moist, sweet, and bright orange in color. In contrast, both white potatoes and yams are "tubers," which are stems, not roots, and are dry, starchy, and generally white or pale yellow in color.

The confusion of true yams (pale tubers) with sweetpotatoes (orange storage roots) started in the 1930s when promoters of Southern-grown sweetpotatoes began using the yam (derived from a West African word, "Inhane," pronounced eenyan) to distinguish their product from the drier, paler sweetpotatoes grown in Northern climates (New Jersey, Maryland, and Virginia). To this day, many grocery stores mislabel one or more variations of actual sweetpotatoes as yams. To avoid confusion, you just need to remember that true yams are paler in color than most sweetpotatoes, rarely sweet, derived from a different part of the plant, and generally not readily available in the United States.

There are three types of sweetpotatoes considered traditional in North American markets—Beauregard, Jewel, and Garnet. These orange-fleshed types have a moist and decidedly sweet quality when cooked. Most of the other kinds of sweetpotatoes sometimes available here are lighter in tone, even white in color and much drier and less sweet in taste than the traditional orange varieties. The most common non-orange types are the Boniato and Asian sweetpotatoes. Asian in this regard is a market catchall term for various rose-skinned, ivory-flesh versions developed in the Far East. When baked, these sweetpotatoes turn yellow with a smooth and semi-dry texture. The traditional orange types are clearly sweeter, much moister, have greater nutritional value (particularly a version of vitamin A) and are strongly preferred by most Americans.

MIKE'S DILEMMA: SWEETPOTATO VERSUS BAGEL

My client Mike overcame his overeating (overgrazing) by transforming his passion for a classic dieter's food that can pile on pounds if overeaten into a passion for sweetpotatoes. When I first met Mike almost two years ago he was not the kind of person who sat down to one or two big meals a day. He was a classic grazer. He preferred a bite here, a nibble there, a snack there, a snack here, and a munch there. This style of eating has many advantages, believe it or not. More frequent meals create more frequent demands on your body, which has to work harder to digest food when it's consumed more often. This, in turn, raises your metabolic rate, the rate at which your body burns energy just to keep you alive and breathing. That can help you lose weight without requiring you to exercise more or eat less.

But one of Mike's challenges was that he often grazed on foods high in calories—sometimes surprisingly so. For example, he often ate several bagels per day. Bagels used to be relatively small, very chewy, and clearly a very low-fat tasty food. In recent years, however, they have grown, with some topping the scale at several ounces—and weighing in at sometimes four hundred to five hundred calories. Mike discovered that sweetpotatoes have many advantages over bagels:

> I work in a mall that has a diverse food court. It includes a great bagel place, but also a grill that bakes potatoes and sweetpotatoes. I found that the warmth and variety of a sweetpotato make them far more filling with far fewer calories. (I make it interesting by adding different sauces, like mustards and barbecue sauces.) I've noticed that if I eat a good-sized sweetpotato, my interest in food is gone for quite a few hours. For someone like me who loves to graze, this is a huge benefit.

Mike, with the help of his very supportive wife, Sheila, found that following the principles in this book allowed them both to lose substantial amounts of weight. Mike has lost forty of the fifty pounds he wanted to lose and his wife lost her total goal of twenty pounds. They've succeeded in maintaining these losses and have found that the substitutions they've made, like the sweetpotatoes for bagels, have left them enjoying their food more than they did before they went on my weight loss program. They now enjoy not only the experience of eating, but also the satisfying feeling of eating constructively, not destructively. That sense of accomplishment feels far better than guilt and self-blame.

TWO DAYS IN MIKE'S LIFE

DAY/DATE: Thursday, February 28
EXERCISE: 35 Min. Treadmill
STEPS: 10,600

Time	Food	Calories	Fat Grams
7:00 A.M.	Skim milk	80	0.0
	2 slices wheat toast	220	0.0
	Jam	30	0.0
	Light peanut butter	75	4.0
8:30 A.M.	Coffee, half & half	30	3.0

Time	Food	Calories	Fat Grams
11:00 A.M.	Hot chocolate	180	1.0
12:30 P.M.	Chicken noodle soup	100	1.0
	Crackers	40	0.0
	Veggie pizza	200	3.0
	Nonfat Yogurt	200	0.0
4:00 P.M.	Skim caramel macchiato	240	1.0
5:00 P.M.	Beef jerky	70	1.0
7:00 P.M.	Boca burger	90	1.5
	Sweetpotato with nonfat cheese	220	0.0
	Pasta/baked beans	190	0.0
	Totals	**1,965**	**15.5**

DAY/DATE: Friday, March 1
EXERCISE: 30 Min. Walk
STEPS: 12,255

Time	Food	Calories	Fat Grams
7:00 A.M.	Coffee, nonfat half & half	40	0.0
8:30 A.M.	Nonfat coffee Coolata	300	0.0
10:30 A.M.	Coffee, half & half	30	3.0
Noon	Black-eyed pea soup	200	0.0
	Crackers	100	3.0
3:00 P.M.	Beef jerky	70	1.0
	Skim milk	120	0.0
5:00 P.M.	Sweetpotato, BBQ sauce	200	0.0
6:30 P.M.	Weight Watchers pasta	240	2.5
	Artichoke with ground turkey breast	160	1.5
	Parmesan cheese	30	1.5
	Skim milk	80	0.0
8:00 P.M.	Coffee/hot chocolate	170	3.0
10:00 P.M.	Nonfat frozen yogurt	200	0.0
	Totals	**1,940**	**15.5**

I've also had clients who developed passions for low-fat soups or cheeseless pizzas. One young client, Rob, began his march to success as a chubby ten-year-old who was four and a half feet tall and weighed 155 pounds. One of Rob's food groups became cheeseless pizza. He either pulled the cheese off his pizza (a Mozzarella-ectomy?) or ordered pizza made without the offending cheese. At least three times a week (sometimes three times a day!), Rob wrote "pizza, no cheese" in his daily eating journal. Eleven years later, Rob now stands more than a foot taller (five feet eleven inches) and weighs nearly the same (165 pounds). If you could grow a foot, you, too, might find your current weight far more acceptable. Unfortunately, almost all seriously over-weight preteens become obese adults. Rob learned to find foods he loved that loved him back and thus avoided the usual pathway from obese preteenager to obese adult.

Cheeseless pizza may not work for you as a primary food, as it did for Rob. Perhaps sweetpotatoes will become a mainstay for you, or broth-based Asian stir-fries or buffalo burgers or turkey hot dogs and beans or some other concoction. The fifty recipes in the final chapter may give you other ideas for lovable foods that love you back. You just have to keep experimenting until you find those lovable foods that bring you comfort, joy, and interest and that keep you healthy. The *Wellspring Plan* works with pleasurable healthy foods, not with diets and deprivation.

Step 5: Move to Lose

STEVE SILVA'S TEARS OF JOY told the story. The ordeal was over. Steve had just completed his heroic assault on the world record for the vertical mile. He had raced up and down the Eiffel Tower seven and a half times, covering a heart-thumping 9,127 steps in two hours, two minutes, and fifty-four seconds.

Steve had finished just one and a half minutes shy of the world record. "I wasn't crying because I didn't make it," said a smiling Steve a few minutes later. "I was just so glad to finish!" By finishing, Steve Silva achieved a much longer climb than the Eiffel Tower. Eight years prior to that moment, Steve weighed 435 pounds. A thirty-nine-year-old high school teacher, he had lost one hundred pounds six different times, only to gain it all back—and more—each time. Steve had ankle problems that made jogging and some other forms of exercise impossible. So he decided to climb stairs. Steve lost 245 pounds (down to a trim and powerful 190 pounds) by climbing up and down thirty thousand steps a week.

Steve said his weight still fluctuates, but now "I eat more, but more veggies. I've learned to have more undereating weeks than overeating weeks." He advises others to "make some reasonable changes; don't expect miracles." This is good advice from a man who has had more experience than almost anyone with life's ups and downs.

Exercise Facts and Fictions

How much do you know about exercising? Most weight controllers accept its importance, but confusions about it are very common. Please take the following "Exercise Test," and use it to evaluate the status of your current knowledge.

EXERCISE TEST		
Circle the best answer for each question.		
1. Exercise doesn't promote weight loss as much as most people think; it takes a lot of exercise to burn off a few calories.	TRUE	FALSE
2. Sit-ups can help you lose fat from the midsection of your body.	TRUE	FALSE
3. Swimming does not help people lose weight.	TRUE	FALSE
4. Overweight people do not have underactive metabolisms.	TRUE	FALSE
5. Increasing daily activities (such as climbing more stairs and walking farther from parking places) does not help people lose weight.	TRUE	FALSE
6. Running three miles burns the same number of calories as walking those three miles.	TRUE	FALSE
7. Women and men burn the same number of calories when they do the same activities.	TRUE	FALSE
8. Jogging five miles per day every day of the week is the ideal exercise regimen for most people.	TRUE	FALSE
9. Exercise can increase appetite.	TRUE	FALSE
10. Exercise cannot affect bones and posture.	TRUE	FALSE
11. If you exercise at the level of your maximum heart rate for more than five minutes, you may die.	TRUE	FALSE
12. It is impossible to maintain the same level of cardiovascular fitness in your sixties that you had when you were in your twenties.	TRUE	FALSE
13. Weightlifting is appropriate for people under fifty, but it presents many risks, especially for those who are older.	TRUE	FALSE
14. Exercising can improve cholesterol levels.	TRUE	FALSE
15. Exercise can improve resting metabolic rate.	TRUE	FALSE

The Exercise Test: Answers and Explanations

1. FALSE. *Exercise* does *promote weight loss at least as much as most people think.* First, you expend significant amounts of calories during the exercise itself. For example, a fast walk for about forty minutes burns off two hundred calories. Second, you expend calories after the walk stops. That is, to replenish the energy consumed during exercise, the body must work harder than it does when it is resting. This increases metabolism. Metabolism is the energy expended by the body to maintain itself (for example, through breathing, digestion, and excretion). Metabolism (or metabolic rate) may remain higher than normal for up to twenty-four hours after exercising. This means that the energy expended by exercising may increase substantially throughout the rest of the day after the exercise is completed. This increase in energy expenditure may amount to doubling the initial amount of calories burned off during the exercise. Third, energy expended during the exercise and by elevating metabolism accumulates day by day, week by week. For example, the forty-minute fast walk, if completed every day, may amount to as much as one pound lost per week. That's fifty pounds per year. Fourth, exercising helps reinforce commitment to weight control. When you exercise, you might think, *Why am I out here sweating when I could be home sleeping?* You may then remind yourself, *I'm out here because I want to control my weight, to look good, to be healthy. I'm here because I'm taking charge of this thing.*

2. FALSE. *Sit-ups* cannot *help you lose fat from your stomach (midsection).* "Spot reduction" simply does not work. Your body takes fat supplies from places that it is directed to by your hormones and genetics. However, sit-ups can improve muscle tone. This could allow you to improve your posture and the appearance of your midsection. You can do this without consciously holding in your stomach. In addition, the improvement in muscle tone from sit-ups and related "crunches" can decrease back problems. When you improve muscle tone in the front and sides of your body, you place less pressure on your back (particularly lower back). Since 80 to 90% of adult Americans develop some back problems (and even a higher percentage of obese people develop these problems), the benefits of sit-ups and crunches are clear.

3. FALSE. *Swimming* can *help people lose weight.* The biological reality is that any energy expenditure can help you lose weight. Swimming places very little strain on the back, the knees, and other weak parts of the body. If you swim approximately twenty yards per minute,

you will expend approximately one hundred calories in about twenty-five minutes. If you sit down for twenty-five minutes, you'll expend approximately twenty-five calories—that is, about 20% of the calories burned when swimming at that slow pace. If you swim at fifty yards per minute, for example, you'll expend one hundred calories in about eight minutes. That's about ten times more calories burned than by sitting.

4. FALSE. *Some overweight people* do *have underactive metabolisms.* Metabolic rates vary just as all biological functions do. Some people are very efficient and expend relatively few calories to keep themselves functioning. Other people are much more inefficient and expend far more calories to keep themselves breathing, digesting, and staying alive. Exercise can increase metabolic rates.

5. FALSE. *Increasing daily activities (such as climbing more stairs and parking farther from stores—causing more walking)* can *help you lose weight.* Any expenditure of energy can help promote weight loss. When you expend more energy than you take in, you lose weight. You expend energy every minute of your life. If you are sitting down or watching television, you expend about 1.5 calories per minute. As soon as you stand up, you burn 20% more calories per minute. When you start moving around a little bit, you burn about three times as many calories per minute compared to sitting. If you start running, energy expenditure goes up to ten times as much as sitting. Table 6.1 makes this point more specifically. Compare calories expended for lying down to standing to walking fast (four miles per hour). You can see that even shopping can help you expend substantial amounts of energy, but more vigorous activities like climbing hills or running dramatically increase expenditures.

Recently one of my newer clients came to a session eager to report on her increase in exercise. She joined an aerobics class and began going to it three times per week. She also discussed her other activities. It turns out she also began gardening recently. She spent a few minutes calculating the number of calories expended during a recent weekend's gardening. She gardened for approximately four hours on both Saturday and Sunday of that weekend. Based on her weight and the calories expended per minute in those activities, calculations showed that she burned approximately 1,200 calories per day by gardening on both Saturday and Sunday. In contrast, her low-impact aerobics class probably resulted in an expenditure of only three hundred calories per class. This means that one afternoon's gardening accounted for greater

TABLE 6.1 CALORIES SPENT PER MINUTE: SITTING VS. STANDING VS. MOVING				
Activity	Weight (pounds)			
	150	200	250	300
Sitting or Lying Down	1.5	2.0	2.5	3.0
Standing Quietly	1.8	2.4	3.0	3.6
Walking Fast (4mph)	6.2	8.2	10.3	12.3
Basketball	9.5	12.6	15.8	18.9
Bicycling				
• (at 5.5mph)	4.4	5.8	7.3	8.7
• (at 9.4mph)	6.8	9.01	1.3	13.5
Canoeing (leisure)	3.0	4.0	5.0	6.0
Chopping Wood	5.9	7.8	9.8	11.7
Cleaning House	4.1	5.4	6.8	8.1
Climbing Hills	8.3	11.0	13.8	16.5
Cooking	3.2	4.2	5.3	6.3
Dancing (slow)	3.5	4.6	5.8	6.9
Dancing (fast)	6.9	9.2	11.5	13.8
Fishing	4.2	5.6	7.0	8.4
Football	9.0	12.0	15.0	18.0
Golf	5.9	7.8	9.8	11.7
Horseback Riding (trot)	7.5	10.0	12.5	15.0
Ironing	3.3	4.4	5.5	6.6
Mopping Floor	4.1	5.4	6.8	8.1
Mowing	7.7	10.2	12.8	15.3
Painting House	5.3	7.0	8.8	10.5
Racquetball	14.4	19.2	25.0	28.8
Raking	3.8	5.0	6.3	7.5
Running				
• 9 min/mile	13.2	17.6	22.0	26.4
• 12 min/mile	9.2	12.2	15.3	18.3
Shopping	4.1	5.4	6.8	8.1
Skiing (downhill)	7.5	10.0	12.5	15.0

TABLE 6.1 (CONTINUED)				
Activity	**Weight (pounds)**			
	150	**200**	**250**	**300**
Swimming				
• Backstroke	11.5	15.4	19.3	23.1
• Breaststroke	11.1	14.8	18.5	22.2
• Crawl (fast)	10.7	14.2	17.8	21.3
• Crawl (slow)	8.7	11.6	14.5	17.4
Table Tennis	4.7	6.2	7.8	9.3
Tennis	7.5	10.0	12.5	15.0
Volleyball	3.5	4.6	5.8	6.9
Walking				
• 3mph	4.7	6.2	7.8	9.3
• 4mph	6.2	8.2	10.3	12.3
Weeding (gardening)	5.0	6.6	8.3	9.9

expenditure of energy than all three aerobics classes in that week! She was amazed. She had lost three pounds that week and had attributed that substantial weight loss to the aerobics classes. Her gardening actually accounted for much more of the weight loss than did the aerobics classes. The lesson here is that whenever you have the opportunity to move, take it.

6. FALSE. *Running three miles burns approximately 50% more calories than walking those three miles.* A study published in 2004 by Dr. Cameron Hall and other exercise physiologists at Syracuse University confirmed this somewhat surprising assertion. When you walk, you move almost exclusively in a horizontal plane, covering distance from your starting point to your finishing point. When you run, you also move in a vertical plane. You're actually jumping a little bit every time you take a step. Just try jumping up and down for a minute and you'll see how much extra energy it takes to contract those big leg muscles. Running also provides the advantages of expending energy in a lot less time and may produce a longer-lasting increase in metabolic rate for several hours or so. Walking has the very substantial advantages, however, of being less painful to do, requiring lower levels of fitness to do, and also producing fewer injuries to knees and backs than running. I have had quite a few clients who lost a lot of weight using running as their primary exercise. I have had many more clients lose weight using

walking as their primary exercise. For example, one of my clients lost 250 pounds doing no other exercise than fast walking (approximately forty-five minutes per day).

7. FALSE. *Since most men weigh considerably more than most women, women and men usually do* not *burn the same number of calories when they do the same activities.* So, if a man and a woman weighed the same amount, they would burn approximately the same number of calories doing the same activities. For example, a 154-pound person would take ten minutes to expend one hundred calories when running a twelve-minute mile—regardless of whether that person was a man or a woman. A 128-pound person would take twelve minutes, running at that same pace, to burn one hundred calories.

8. FALSE. *Jogging five miles per day every day of the week is* not *the ideal exercise regimen for most people.* Jogging is a wonderful form of exercise. It is efficient and it produces many benefits. However, jogging pounds the knees, jars the hips, crunches the spinal column, and can contribute to a variety of back problems. The risk of knee, back, hip, and other problems increases substantially if you jog more than five days per week. These orthopedic risks also increase substantially when you jog for more than thirty minutes per outing. Since almost everyone would take quite a bit more than thirty minutes to jog five miles, the combination of jogging five miles plus jogging seven out of seven days creates a substantial risk for injury. Overweight people in particular would be ill-advised to attempt such a regimen. Excess weight creates excess pounding on the knees and increases the likelihood of foot, hip, and back problems. Walking seven days per week, on the other hand, would create fewer such problems.

9. TRUE. *Exercise can increase appetite; but mild to moderate exercise can actually* decrease *appetite.* For example, most people find they desire food less if they exercise ten, fifteen, twenty, and even sixty minutes. However, exercising for several hours often *increases* appetite. You can prevent this increase in appetite by eating or drinking beverages with calories during extended periods of exercise. Liquids are easiest to digest during exercise and carbohydrates are also relatively easy to digest. For example, fruit juices and fruit make good appetite suppressants during extended exercise.

10. FALSE. *Exercise* can *affect bones and posture.* After about age thirty-five, bone mass (sometimes called bone density) gradually decreases. This bone loss can lead to osteoporosis—the weakening of your bones—causing them to break easily. Exercise preserves bone

mass or density. Consider what happens when adults stay in bed (for example, during illness or hospitalization). They typically lose as much bone mass in two weeks as they would normally lose in a year. Studies have shown that exercising regularly can actually build bone in older people. One such study showed an increase in bone mass in a group of women whose average age was eighty-one.

11. FALSE. *You can exercise at the level of your maximum heart rate for far more than five minutes without any concern about dying.* You could actually survive at your maximum heart rate for many days. This principle holds unless you have a heart condition.

12. FALSE. *It is very possible to maintain the same level of cardiovascular fitness in your sixties that you had when you were in your twenties.* Remember your hunter-gatherer ancestry. Hunter-gatherers maintained high levels of activity throughout their lifetimes. People in industrialized countries maintain high levels of activity during childhood (at least most people do), but they become more and more sedentary as they get older. Inactivity begets weakness; weakness begets injuries and more weakness. Studies show that regular aerobic exercise can maintain cardiovascular fitness and can even reverse some of the damage done by sedentary living. For example, in a recent study, nineteen men and women in their sixties exercised aerobically for about one hour three times per week. After two months, their resting metabolic rates increased by about 10% (on average), virtually eliminating the decline in resting metabolic rate caused naturally by the aging process. Aerobic capacities, or fitness levels, can also improve radically with persistent exercising. Many reports testify to the remarkable conditioning of runners and other committed athletes who were measured in their youths and then again in old age. Very few declines in aerobic conditioning occurred for these athletes. As people grow older, reflexes slow down and some decreases in flexibility seem almost inevitable. Cardiovascular fitness, however, can be maintained at very high levels. Sixty-year-olds can, indeed, have cardiovascular systems like twenty-year-olds (see Table 6.2).

13. FALSE. *Weightlifting is very appropriate for people of all ages.* With proper supervision, even ninety-year-olds can benefit from weightlifting. For example, a study with ten ninety-year-olds had them lift weights with their legs for ten to twenty minutes, three times per week. After eight weeks, they could lift three times more weight than they could prior to beginning weightlifting. Two of the nonagenarians gave up their canes after just eight weeks of lifting.

14. TRUE. *Exercise* can *improve cholesterol levels.* Some evidence suggests that regular exercising can increase the level of HDL or "good cholesterol."

15. TRUE. *Exercise* can *improve resting metabolic rate.* Metabolic rate refers to the rate at which your body uses (metabolizes) energy when you are resting. Your body uses quite a bit of energy even when you rest in order to digest food, keep you breathing, and so on. Studies with both animals and humans show that your body slows down your metabolic rate when you start eating less than usual. This would allow you to survive during food shortages when the hunting and gathering is not going well. If you exercise regularly, however, your body reacts as if everything is okay. If you are moving around a lot, then your body "knows" you must not be starving. So, every day you exercise your body will keep your metabolic rate high. This important effect means that on days that you exercise, your body will expend more energy all day, thus allowing you to lose weight more easily than if you hadn't exercised that day.

Benefits of Exercising

The "Exercise Test" makes it clear that exercising is critical for effective weight control. Steven Blair also made this point with his "Exercise Quiz," published in *The Weight Control Digest*. You may improve your commitment to exercising if you understand the many ways exercise can affect you. While you know exercise can improve your ability to control your weight, do you know how exercising can affect you as you grow older? Table 6.2 makes critical comparisons between the fit person you can become versus the sedentary person you must stop being in order to succeed. Fitness provides increasing and more dramatic benefits as you get older.

The exercise test and the comparison of fit versus sedentary women illustrate some of the many benefits of exercising. The following list describes even more.

Exercise can:

1. Increase weight loss
2. Improve maintenance of weight losses
3. Improve stress management
4. Improve the quality of sleep

TABLE 6.2 ONLY THE FIT STAY YOUNG: CHANGES IN WOMEN'S BODIES	
The Fit Woman	**The Sedentary Woman**
TWENTIES	
She retains the strength, stamina and flexibility of her teen years. Her leanness allows the definition of her muscles to show through. Late in this decade her bone strength may reach its peak. If she continues regular weight-bearing exercises, consumes plenty of calcium-rich foods, and gets adequate caloric intake, her bones will stay healthy for years to come. A lot of time spent outdoors without adequate sun protection will cause her skin to begin to freckle and develop very fine lines.	She may look great, but physical changes are already beginning to take place that could have far-reaching effects. Her aerobic capacity begins to decline at the rate of 1% per year. After age twenty-five, muscle mass can decrease by an average of 5% every decade. Metabolism begins to drop at a rate of 2% per year, which will translate into increasingly higher body-fat percentages. Any fat added now will be distributed evenly throughout her body. She will begin to experience tightness in her hips.
THIRTIES	
She looks and feels as fit as in her twenties. She's agile and coordinated, with a lean, defined physique, thanks to well-developed muscles and below-average body fat, and her aerobic capacity—the ability to transport oxygen throughout the body—is better than ever. She will, however, begin to experience an unavoidable decline in the number of fast-twitch muscles, which are responsible for quick reaction time and for high-intensity activities like sprinting. If bone strength has not yet peaked, it will by age thirty-five.	She will begin to feel her age in terms of muscle strength, particularly in her arms and legs. This is because her muscle fibers are starting to atrophy, and her muscle mass will continue to decline at a rate of about 6.6% each decade from here on out. She feels stiffer, as elastin is lost from her muscles. She could have as much as 33% body fat, most of it concentrated in her hips and thighs. Along with that of her active peers, her sexual responsiveness reaches a peak—but she may not have the energy to enjoy it.
FORTIES	
She remains as energetic and flexible as ever, with excellent aerobic stamina. Because of an inevitable decline in metabolism, however, she may have a tendency to put on some fat—particularly in hips and thighs. But her high muscle-to-fat ratio keeps her calorie-burning capacity up, and this, along with continued aerobic exercise, will counteract this tendency to gain fat, keeping her at about 11% body fat. Although she experiences some compression of the vertebrae in her back, strong muscles keep her stomach relatively flat, her back supple.	She is by now 15% weaker than she was in her thirties, and the decline will be even more dramatic past age forty-five. Her shoulders appear narrower as muscle mass decreases in her upper back. The disks between her vertebrae begin to compress, so that with time she will be one to one and a half inches shorter and her stomach will distend as the distance between her ribs and pelvis decreases. She has lost about 40% of the range of motion in her hips and may develop varicose veins.

TABLE 6.2 (CONTINUED)	
The Fit Woman	**The Sedentary Woman**
FIFTIES	
She has maintained every aspect of fitness. Her age shows only in her percentage of body fat, which continues to increase slightly—it's probably up to about 24% now. Gravity may start to take its toll on her body, and she may feel some wear and tear in her joints due to years of activity. She may want to rethink her workouts, switching to lower-impact activity—swimming or walking, for example.	She has poor posture due to the continued drop in flexibility and muscle strength. She slouches forward and has a protruding stomach and overarched lower back. All the repercussions of inadequate aerobic activity begin to kick in: Her blood pressure rises; she becomes more susceptible to diabetes and heart attacks. Now body fat begins to settle around her middle, her skin wrinkles and is tugged downward by gravity.
SIXTIES	
She has strong, flexible muscles and plenty of stamina. Despite the effect menopause has on estrogen production, her bones are strong thanks in part to the weight-bearing exercises and strength training she's done all her life (although hormone replacement may be necessary). Her target heart rate will be about 115 beats per minute (down thirty or forty bpm from her twenties). But because aerobic exercise has kept her heart strong, she remains able to pump healthy amounts of blood. She has about 26% body fat.	She is two or three inches shorter by now and may have developed osteoporosis, partly because she has not done the weight-bearing exercise that keeps bones strong. Her breasts begin to sag in earnest and her waist widens even more. Her heart is 10 to 15% weaker than it was when she was twenty and measurable changes in her immune system increase her risk of developing cancer and certain infections. Wrinkles are now creases, and skin is dry.
SEVENTIES	
She can work and play almost as hard as she did thirty years ago. Only a slight increase in body fat—amplified by the earth's pull—reveals her age, along with deeper creases in her face and a drier look to her skin due to a decline in oil production that occurs after menopause.	She is in failing health as high blood pressure, brittle bones, and unhealthy blood cholesterol levels leave her vulnerable to a host of serious diseases. Her flexibility, strength, and stamina are about nil, and she may have developed the classic "dowager's hump." She has wrinkles in her cheeks, and her mouth turns down, so she appears as unhappy as she probably feels.

(Source: *self* Magazine, September 1992)

5. Improve digestion
6. Enhance self-esteem
7. Improve resistance to illnesses
8. Help you feel energized
9. Promote better digestion and bowel functioning
10. Tone muscles
11. Provide more definition to muscles
12. Reduce blood pressure
13. Reduce tension
14. Improve flexibility
15. Build strength
16. Promote greater endurance
17. Decrease the negative effects of aging
18. Decrease menstrual cramping
19. Increase metabolic rate
20. Enhance coordination
21. Improve posture
22. Decrease back problems and pain
23. Decrease resting heart rate
24. Strengthen bones and joints
25. Improve reaction time
26. Strengthen the heart
27. Prevent heart disease
28. Improve cholesterol levels
29. Prevent osteoporosis (weakness of the bones)
30. Decrease the risk of cancer (particularly colon cancer)
31. Improve abilities to relax more quickly
32. Decrease depression
33. Increase emotional stability
34. Improve quality of thinking
35. Improve ability to stay warm in colder climates
36. Improve ability to tolerate warmer climates
37. Improve agility
38. Improve body image
39. Increase endorphins (internally produced opiates that improve feelings of well-being and mood)
40. Decrease constipation
41. Improve social life (for example, by meeting new people during exercising)
42. Improve athletic performance

43. Increase life span
44. Increase feelings of control or mastery
45. Improve rosiness of complexion
46. Decrease appetite
47. Provide balance in life
48. Increase self-awareness
49. Provide time to think, gain perspective, and solve problems more effectively
50. Promote self-actualization

This is a rather convincing list, isn't it? Many of the benefits of exercise pertain directly to weight control. Changes in muscles, bones, fat, and attitude can all affect success at weight control. In fact, some studies of successful weight controllers show that virtually 100% become frequent exercisers. Some of these studies included people who lost fifty pounds or more and maintained it for more than five years. On average, these master weight controllers walk briskly for one hour per day—every day. Only 20% of Americans over twenty-five years old exercise at least twice per week. This also means that most Americans, the sedentary ones, place themselves at unnecessarily high risk for developing cancer, as described in the story below.

Can Exercise Prevent Cancer?

Seventy-five years ago, two Minnesota physicians noticed that most of their patients who developed cancer led sedentary lives. They also noticed that patients who were farmers rarely developed cancer. They speculated that hard work and physical activity might prevent cancer. They compared cancer rates among various occupations. As they expected, cancer rates decreased as physical activity increased.

More recent research has supported the idea that exercising regularly can prevent cancer. A study of thirteen thousand people conducted by the Institute for Aerobics Research in Dallas used the treadmill test to measure fitness levels and then track cancer rates over eight years. They found that the men who were least fit had more than four times the overall cancer rates than the most-fit men. The least-fit women had sixteen times higher death rates due to cancer than the most-fit women.

Exercising probably decreases colon cancer, breast cancer, and possibly prostate cancer. Cancer of the colon is the second leading cause of death (next to lung cancer) in the United States. Fifty thousand Americans die each year from cancer of the colon. Twenty-one of twenty-seven recent studies have found that as activity increases, rates of colon cancer decrease.

Exercise may prevent colon cancer by increasing the speed at which waste products get through the colon. Greater physical activity leads to greater mobility in the intestines, as well. Also, greater physical activity might affect some biochemical agents that promote increased speed of digestion. It follows that the less time waste products spend in the colon, the less time those waste products that contain cancer-causing substances (carcinogens) spend in the body.

An important study on breast cancer involved more than five thousand women who graduated from college between 1925 and 1981. The women who had been college athletes had about half the risk of breast cancer compared to non-athletes. Another study of twenty-five thousand women in the state of Washington showed that those who had worked in physically active jobs had much lower incidences of breast cancer than those who had sedentary occupations. Exercising may prevent breast cancer because it lowers estrogen levels.

Research on more than seventeen thousand Harvard alumni showed that among men over age seventy, those who had remained most active had much lower incidences of prostate cancer than the least active men. However, the "most active" men expended more than three thousand calories per week in walking, climbing stairs, and playing sports compared to the least active men. The high level of activity it takes to expend these three thousand calories may decrease levels of the male hormone, testosterone. Lowering this hormone may decrease the risk of prostate cancer.

Frequent exercisers tend to have other habits associated with the decreased risk of cancer. For example, frequent exercisers smoke less and eat lower-fat diets than sedentary people. However, most of the studies on exercise and cancer did eliminate these factors when analyzing the effects of exercise. In other words, those studies found exercising reduces risks of getting cancer regardless of the effects of diet and smoking. It seems safe to conclude that exercising regularly can prevent certain types of cancer.

How to Move to Lose

Is it advisable to exercise every day? Is it advisable to exercise for twenty minutes per day? Forty? Sixty? What kinds of activities produce optimal results for weight controllers: aerobic exercise, weightlifting, or a combination of both? Do everyday activities like walking to the bus or shopping help people lose weight?

The American College of Sports Medicine (ACSM), which consists of many of the world's premier experts on exercising, has provided recommendations to answer these questions. Its most recent set of recommendations has become accepted around the world as the basis for developing safe and effective exercising patterns. Let's review answers to commonly asked questions by considering five aspects of exercising and the ACSM recommendations that pertain to them:

Frequency of Exercise. Since exercising is so critical to weight control, I strongly encourage each of my clients to exercise every single day. This exercise can vary from walking to swimming to playing racquetball. If you become accustomed to exercising in some form every day, you will lose more weight and maintain that weight loss more effectively. ACSM recommends six days per week to lose weight. Because of the many benefits for weight control, however, I recommend placing an even greater emphasis on exercise.

Setting a *daily* exercise goal may well improve your consistency as it limits the excuses you can use to avoid exercising. If you adopted a five-day-per-week goal, you could easily say to yourself, *Today is the day I won't exercise. I'll exercise tomorrow.* This kind of thinking allows for many reasons to skip days. Have you said to yourself, *I don't feel like it today* or *I don't have time today*? If you commit thoroughly to a daily goal, it makes it more difficult to allow yourself to postpone this critical aspect of your well-being. Some of my clients have used a wonderful expression to capture this: "not exercising is not an option." Remember, you are pursuing something other than a general improvement in your health. You are combating biological forces that are dead set against weight loss. This takes extraordinary effort and commitment.

Mode of Exercise: Steps Matter Most! When I was growing up in Brooklyn in the 1950s, jogging didn't really exist. If you saw a man running down the street, you knew someone else was chasing him. The term "running shoes" also did not exist. The idea of spending as much money for "running shoes" as some people spend on a set of tires still amazes me.

The world has changed a great deal in the past fifty years. Options for exercising are everywhere. Health clubs are no longer places for fanatics. They are commonplace in many communities—especially in urban centers. Almost everyone has not only heard of running shoes— everyone owns at least one pair. Joggers run everywhere. Exercising has become part of everyday life.

But which options produce the best outcomes for weight controllers? My clients ask about the benefits of stair-climbing machines versus treadmills. People wonder about exercise equipment they can buy for their homes versus equipment in health clubs. Personal trainers have become another addition to the possibilities for exercising.

Research shows that three elements of exercising seem particularly helpful: convenience, appeal, and social aspects. First, *convenience* affects exercising. If you join a health club twenty miles from your home or twenty miles from work, would you really use it regularly enough? Most people would not. In fact, many health clubs advertise as aggressively as possible to get people to join. The clubs realize that most people will not use the facilities even after signing up and paying for membership; their greatest profit comes from people who join and then disappear! Certainly walking, jogging, and in-home exercising are very convenient for most people. When looking at health clubs, consider joining one that requires minimal transportation. If you can find one next door to your job or within walking distance from home, it may be the best buy for you.

Second, the *appeal* of an exercise routine affects your use of it. Do you like walking? Or do you prefer a more social and musical activity like aerobics classes? Perhaps if you can make a game of your exercising, you would pursue it more effectively. Some people like racquetball and tennis because they enjoy the competition and camaraderie of those sports. You can also make your exercising as enjoyable as possible. Research shows that people who walk or jog exercise more vigorously and consistently if they use a Walkman-type radio or CD player or iPod. Setting up a treadmill at home is an art form in and of itself. It helps to use earphones (wireless earphones are especially good) connected to the television and to a CD player to provide a variety of distractions. Many people also exercise at home in front of a DVD player while watching rented movies.

Finally, *social* aspects of exercise can affect consistency. If you can walk with a friend or spouse, you may find walking far more enjoyable than solitary journeys. The "loneliness of the long-distance runner" can make it difficult to remain enthusiastic about exercising on your own. In contrast, some people like the time alone that exercise provides. I have heard many people say, "Let me run on that tomorrow morning." These runners use their jogging time to solve problems. Problem solving goes remarkably well when phones aren't ringing and people aren't knocking on the door. If you are one of those people who enjoys the company of others while exercising, social sports such as golf and bowling add an important dimension to exercising.

My clients tend to prefer treadmills over exercycles. The people who own treadmills seem to use them more frequently. Unfortunately, *Consumer Reports'* engineers found that most lower-cost treadmills do not work very well. They tend to be noisy and break down regularly. You might have to pay around $1,000 for a high-quality, relatively quiet and reliable piece of equipment that should last for many years.

While exercise DVDs provide tremendous convenience—both in location and finances—they often contain inappropriate information and some offer potentially dangerous advice. Physiologists Nicki Euloff and David Thomas evaluated the ten top-selling videos. These experts found that four of the videos contained as little as five minutes of aerobic exercise. Two contained none at all! Several of the videos do not include enough warm-up time. *All* of the videos studied included exercise against which the experts strongly advised. These exercises included "ballistic stretching without adequate warm-up." Ballistic stretching is sudden, jerky movements designed to increase flexibility. "Static stretching" is vastly preferred because it increases flexibility by slowly stretching a muscle and holding it in that position for several seconds. Ballistic stretching can tear or strain muscles very easily. Many of the videos also included overextension of certain regions of the spine and knee joints. Luckily, more recent videos have improved somewhat. For example, Kathy Smith has created several safer and more appropriate videos (*Kathy Smith: Starting Out* and *Kathy Smith's Winning Workout*).

Steps for Success. The problem with excess weight in America, and most likely in your life, reflects our culture's lack of basic movement compared to most other countries in the world. For example, at least 40% of trips in urban areas of Austria, Denmark, the Netherlands, and Sweden are made by bicycle or feet. People travel by bike or walk for at least 30% of their urban trips in France, Germany, and Switzerland.

Here in the land of plenty, however, only 10% of city travel occurs outside of cars, buses, or trains. In the relatively newer cities in the United States, like Los Angeles, Atlanta, and Dallas, less than 5% of trips involve biking or walking. Compare that percentage to those in the older cities in Europe, like London (35%) and Amsterdam (47%).

Ten thousand steps a day is the most commonly recommended goal. (And don't forget my advice in Chapter 1: Get a pedometer!) A recent study found that thirty minutes a day of moderate activity results in about eight thousand steps, a total that includes the three thousand to five thousand steps per day that most adults accumulate without even attempting to increase their activity levels. At Wellspring Academy—California, the boarding school I helped develop for Wellspring, students average 14,500 steps. Those students lose about three pounds per week. At our Wellspring Camps, campers lose weight even more rapidly, averaging four pounds per week, and average as much as twenty thousand steps per day in our adventure camps (camps that involve quite a few very active off-site camping trips). Of course, the food at these sites is exactly the type recommended in this book, with very little outside foods creeping in around the edges. In a less well-controlled world, like the one in which you find yourself, you can aim for ten thousand steps (or more) as your initial goal and see how it affects your weight control program.

The following chart shows the impact of achieving a goal like ten thousand steps per day. Dr. Ross Andersen and his colleagues at the Johns Hopkins University School of Medicine found that their "High Steppers" reached activity goals like ten thousand steps per day 79% of the weeks in a one-year follow-up period. These High Steppers had lost an average of twenty pounds in a weight-control program prior to beginning the follow-up phase. "Low Steppers" who had also lost about twenty pounds during the weight loss program only reached the activity goals in 19% of the weeks during the follow-up. You can see the dramatic differences in weight change at the end of the follow-up period that clearly favored the High Steppers. You've got to move to lose and to keep the weight off.

Intensity of Exercise. Intensity refers to how hard your body works during a certain length of time. More intensive exercise means that your body works harder for the fifteen or thirty or forty-five minutes during which you exercise. Intensity varies depending on your level of conditioning or fitness. For example, world-class marathoners can run three eight-minute miles in a row and fail to break a sweat. For

CHART 6.1: HIGH STEPPERS VS. LOW STEPPERS

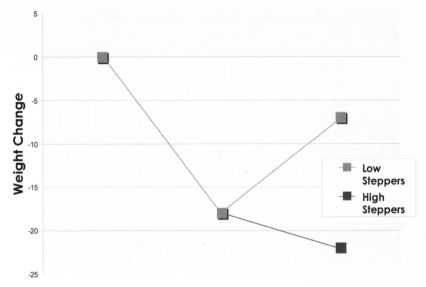

Time (baseline, post-treatment,1-year follow-up)

Dramatic differences between weight controllers who reached their exercise goals for one year on 79% of the weeks after a treatment program ended ("High Steppers") versus those who reached their exercise goals in only 19% of the weeks ("Low Steppers"). Based on a study by Dr. Ross Andersen and his colleagues (*Journal of the American Medical Association*, 1999, v. 281, pp. 335–340).

the non-runner's body, this intensity level would be very high. For the world-class marathoner, this intensity is very low.

Intensity of exercise is measured in several ways. The simplest way to measure it involves heart rate. The average resting heart rate of a forty-five-year-old man is about seventy-two beats per minute. During moderate exercise, this increases to 145 beats per minute. Maximum exercise may lead to a heart rate of 175 beats per minute. This man's heart generally pumps about five liters of blood per minute while he is resting. During heavy exercise, his heart pumps about four times that amount of blood (twenty liters) and his breathing rate goes from twelve breaths per minute to forty-three breaths per minute. His systolic blood pressure goes from 120 to 200 (mmHg). These biological changes occur because the body consumes a lot of energy and a lot of oxygen when it works hard. The muscle cells consume energy in the form of stored sugar (glycogen, glucose) as well as fats. The consumption of this energy requires oxygen, which is also used quickly during intensive exercise.

Your heart has a maximum capability for pumping blood and helping your body function during intensive exercising. You can actually sustain your maximum heart rate for many hours and perhaps many days. However, this maximum rate is considered an upper limit from which you can judge the intensity of your exercising. Subtract your age from 220 to calculate your maximum heart rate. If you are forty years old, your maximum heart rate is 180 beats per minute (220 - 40 = 180). When you exercise at high intensity levels (close to your maximum heart rate), you become exhausted very quickly. You also increase your risk of injury through sprains and strains. In contrast, when you exercise at 60 to 80% of your maximum heart rate (your "training heart rate"), you stress your system in a positive way. This level of overloading your cardiovascular system can actually increase your heart's ability to pump blood throughout your body. By exercising at this recommended training heart rate, your muscles become increasingly efficient at extracting oxygen from your blood. This increase in efficiency takes time. It usually takes several weeks of fairly frequent exercise to improve efficiency at extracting oxygen from the blood and strengthening your heart. Gradually, however, anyone who exercises at this training rate enough becomes an increasingly fit individual.

Sometimes the term "aerobic capacity" is used to describe this type of fitness. Aerobic simply means involving oxygen. When you become aerobically fit, you increase your heart's ability to pump oxygenated blood through your body and you increase the efficiency of your muscles at extracting oxygen from your blood. The more fit you are, the more oxygen and fuel (glucose, fat) you can get into your muscles quickly. This allows your muscles to work hard for long periods of time without producing feelings of exhaustion.

The most important rule of thumb about intensity of exercise is this: keep the intensity low enough to allow yourself to exercise for at least thirty minutes per session. Many people, like the birthday boy in the personal testimony below, make the mistake of exercising too intensely for their current fitness levels. As a result, they become tired and find exercise painful after only a few minutes. If you jog at a slow pace (twelve-minute miles), you expend about ten calories per minute. If you walk at a moderate pace (twenty-minute miles), you expend about five calories per minute. Weight control depends on total amount of energy expended. If you weigh two hundred pounds and can only jog for five minutes at a nine-minute-mile pace, you expend only about 88 calories during that exercise session. On the other hand, if you can walk for thirty minutes at the moderate twenty-minute-mile pace, you would expend more than twice that amount of calories. You expend more energy by exercising for a longer period of time at the lower intensity level. That's what matters most for weight control. *Expend energy using an intensity that you can tolerate.*

WHICH IS BETTER—EXERCISE OR GETTING YOUR TEETH DRILLED?

For my birthday this year my wife bought me a week of private lessons at the local health club. Though still in great shape from when I was on the varsity chess team in high school, I decided it was a good idea to go ahead and try it. I called and made reservations with someone named Tanya, who said she was a twenty-six-year-old aerobics instructor and athletic clothing model. My wife seemed very pleased with how enthusiastic I was to get started.

DAY 1: They suggest I keep this "exercise diary" to chart my progress this week. Started the morning at six A.M. Tough to get up, but worth it when I arrived at the health club and Tanya was waiting for me. She's something of a goddess, with blond hair and a dazzling white smile. She showed me the machines and took my pulse after five minutes on the treadmill. She seemed a little alarmed that it was so high, but I think just standing next to her in that outfit of hers added about ten points. Enjoyed watching the aerobics class. Tanya was very encouraging as I did my sit-ups, though my gut was already aching a little from holding it in the whole time I was talking to her. This is going to be *GREAT*.

DAY 2: Took a whole pot of coffee to get me out the door, but I made it. Tanya had me lie on my back and push this heavy iron bar up into the air. Then she put weights on it, for heaven's sake! Legs were a little wobbly on the treadmill, but I made it the full mile. Her smile made it all worth it. Muscles feel *GREAT*.

DAY 3: The only way I can brush my teeth is by laying the toothbrush on the counter and moving my mouth back and forth over it. I am certain that I have developed a hernia in both pectorals. Driving was okay as long as I didn't try to steer. I parked on top of a Volkswagen. Tanya was a little impatient with me and said my screaming was bothering the other club members. The treadmill hurt my chest so I did the stair monster. Why would anyone invent a machine to simulate an activity rendered obsolete by the invention of elevators? Tanya told me regular exercise would make me live longer. I can't imagine anything worse.

DAY 4: Tanya was waiting for me with her vampire teeth in a full snarl. I can't help it if I was half an hour late—it took me that long just to tie my shoes. She wanted me to lift dumbbells. Not a chance, Tanya. The world "dumb" must be in there for a reason. I hid in the men's room until she sent Lars looking for me. As punishment she made me try the rowing machine. It sank.

DAY 5: I hate Tanya more than any human being has ever hated any other human being in the history of the world. If there was any part of my body not in extreme pain, I would hit her with it. She thought it would be a good idea to work on my triceps. Well, I have news for you, Tanya, I don't have triceps. And if you don't want dents in the floor don't hand me any barbells. I refuse to accept responsibility for the damage. YOU went to sadist school. YOU are to blame. The treadmill flung me back into a science teacher, which hurt like crazy. Why couldn't it have been someone softer, like a music teacher, or social studies?

DAY 6: Got Tanya's message on my answering machine, wondering where I am. I lacked the strength to use the TV remote so I watched eleven straight hours of the Weather Channel.

DAY 7: Well, that's the week. Thank God that's over. Maybe next time my wife will give me something a little more fun, like free tooth drilling at the dentist.

If you don't want to end up like this birthday boy, don't overdo it! For a quick check of exercise intensity levels, review the target zones listed in the following table for people ranging in age from twenty to ninety years.

After six months or more of regular exercising, you can exercise up to 85% of your maximum heart rate. However, you do not have to

Age	Target Zone (60–80%, beats/minute)	Maximum Heart Rate (100%)
20	120–160	200
25	117–156	195
30	114–152	190
35	111–148	185
40	108–144	180
45	105–140	175
50	102–136	170
55	99–132	165
60	96–128	160
65	93–124	155
70	90–120	150
75	87–116	145
80	84–112	140
85	81–108	135

TABLE 6.3 — TARGET HEART RATE ZONES FOR EXERCISING TO IMPROVE FITNESS

exercise that hard to stay in excellent condition. To check your heart rate during exercise, take your pulse immediately after you stop exercising:

1. When you stop exercising, place the tips of your first two fingers lightly over one of the blood vessels on your neck (carotid arteries) to the left or right of the center of your throat. Another convenient place to determine your heart rate (or pulse) is the inside of your wrist just below the base of your thumb.
2. Count your pulse for ten seconds and multiply by six.
3. If your pulse (heart rate) is below your target zone, consider exercising a little more intensely next time. If you are above your target zone, exercise a little less intensely the next time. If your pulse falls within your target zone, you are doing fine.

Remember, any exercise, even exercise way below your target zone, helps promote effective weight control and improve cardiovascular fitness. If your intensity level begins to feel too high, you may also find it helpful to check your heart rate to see whether you are in your target zone. You will probably find that you feel quite uncomfortable when you exercise above your target zone. Decreasing your intensity should allow you to exercise for thirty minutes or more.

Many people seek to increase the mass or size of their muscles both for the appearance and to increase their metabolic rates (energy expended by your body when you are resting). Muscle cells consume more calories than fat and than most other tissues, after all. So, the logical thinking goes, if I have more muscle in my body, I can eat more and still lose weight. Unfortunately, the intensity of exercise required to increase muscle mass is very demanding, more demanding than most people realize. You'd probably have to exercise until you produced what is called "muscle failure" (exhaustion of the specific muscle group, feeling that you can't lift any more weight) for many hours per week in order to increase the mass of your muscles. This takes a lot of time and is also quite uncomfortable. Women would have to exercise much more than men to produce this muscle failure because their bodies put up a much stronger fight against gaining muscle mass.

All of the difficulties of increasing muscle mass help explain why professional athletes sometimes take illegal substances (like steroids) and numerous untested (scientifically) supplements in order to increase their strength and the bulk of their muscles. As a weight controller, you'll get far more payoff using your activities and exercises to expend energy instead of to bulk up. If you do things that don't produce discomfort (which exercising to produce muscle failure certainly does) and that you like to do (like walking with your spouse), then you'll be far more likely to maintain this critical aspect of your program.

Duration of Exercise. The American College of Sports Medicine endorses exercise sessions lasting from thirty to sixty minutes. Many people have difficulty maintaining aerobic activities for thirty minutes or more. If you are one of these people, try starting with sessions that last ten or fifteen minutes. Two fifteen-minute sessions of exercise produce about the same benefits as one thirty-minute session. In fact, from a weight-control perspective, you will enjoy better results from frequent exercise for shorter amounts of time compared to one long session.

Some confusing theories exist about the length of exercise sessions. One concerns "fat burning." It suggests that you won't "burn fat" unless you exercise for long periods of time. This assertion is wrong. When you begin exercising, you begin using calories immediately. The energy consumed by your body initially comes from glucose stored in the muscles. As you exercise for longer periods of time, your body begins dipping into its energy reserves (fat). However, your body must replenish the energy supply it uses. This means that when you consume energy in the form of stored glucose from the muscles, your body will use its stored energy supply to replenish the glucose taken from the muscles. It makes no difference whether you exercise for short bursts of ten or fifteen minutes or for longer periods of thirty to sixty minutes per session. You burn fat in both ways.

One of my clients, Ellen, described how she began exercising for very short periods of time. She then gradually extended the duration of her exercise:

> I began exercising for fifteen seconds at a time on my Schwinn Air-Dyne with the oversized seat. I just couldn't seem to stay on that thing for more than a few seconds at a time. Of course, I weighed 340 pounds when I started using it. So, I did fifteen seconds three times a day. Then I was able to do it longer and longer every day. Now, 190 pounds later, I use my Air-Dyne for thirty to forty minutes every morning. Sometimes I go to an aerobics class or do a fast walk instead. But, I exercise every day, sometimes twice a day. It makes me feel reasonably good. Although, I must admit, I would quit it all in a second if I could find some other way of keeping healthy and keeping my weight down. Exercising like I do sure beats the alternative of being so big.

Strength Training (Weightlifting). It is a little-known fact that by age seventy-four about one-third of all men and two-thirds of all women can't lift a gallon of milk (which weighs approximately ten pounds). The average adult loses about six or seven pounds of muscle per decade after that. Most seventy-year-olds have one-third fewer muscle cells than they had at age twenty. Also, the muscle cells of seventy-year-olds are smaller than those of twenty-year-olds. Aging, however, does not cause these declines in muscularity. Disuse and sedentary living cause this weakening of the muscles.

In 1990, the ACSM recognized and emphasized the importance of resistance training more than in any of their previous recommendations. Strength training of moderate intensity (50 to 60% of maximal lifting ability) provides important benefits. The ACSM recommends selecting exercises that incorporate many different body parts and different kinds of movements. They suggest performing lifting exercises continuously, using smooth, slow, and controlled motions. Maintaining good posture when lifting weights also helps avoid injury. Only the body part being exercised while lifting the weight should be in motion during a lift. Other body parts should be at rest and stationary when weightlifting.

Let's review several other critical questions about weightlifting:

How many repetitions? Eight to twelve repetitions improve both strength and endurance. Most exercise experts suggest that if you can lift the weight easily more than twelve times, it is time to add more weight. When you add more weight, go back to eight to twelve repetitions per exercise.

How many sets? The ACSM recommends using eight to ten different kinds of weight lifting exercises per set. A set is a group of exercises completed one time. For example, you might do a set of eight exercise, that include one or two for your arms, some for your midsection, some for your legs, and so on. If you only make time to do one set, you will still strengthen your muscles 70 to 80% as much as you would by doing multiple sets. A full set of eight or ten exercises, including warm-up time, can take as little as fifteen minutes to do.

How many workouts? The ideal strengthening program includes three workouts a week. Squeezing in more than three workouts per week might slow the growth of your muscles. Muscles may need some time off to recover from weight training. Interestingly, you can get about 75% of the maximum improvement available from weightlifting by working out only twice a week. If you don't have much time, even a single strengthening session per week helps far more than none at all. According to one study, a weekly workout can maintain current levels of strength for several months.

Strength training for the legs? People who do aerobic exercises may not need strengthening exercises for the legs. Most aerobic exercises keep leg muscles in good shape. However, strengthening for the legs may improve your ability to run, play sports, or climb stairs. It can also help older people walk longer distances and may prevent knee and hip injuries.

How much is enough? To keep building strength, you must keep increasing the weights you lift. You can maintain a desired level of strength by simply maintaining twelve repetitions for a particular exercise. If you stop weightlifting, your strength will begin to fade within two weeks. After three to five months, you'll be back to where you started.

What's the procedure for weightlifting? Several guidelines can help prevent injuries and maximize the benefits of weightlifting. First, it helps to warm up for a few minutes by walking briskly or jogging in place and then do stretching exercises. Stretch your shoulders, lower back, calves, and front and back of the thighs. Stretch slowly and steadily to the point of tension—not pain—and hold the position for three to thirty seconds. As you get more flexible, you'll be able to hold the positions for thirty seconds; just hold the positions as long as you can at first, even if you can only hold them for three seconds each.

Second, breathe slowly and steadily during weightlifting. Holding your breath while tensing muscles can cause light-headedness and even fainting. Exhale as you either lift the weight or raise your body and inhale as you return to the starting position. Third, perform the repetitions slowly. Each one should take about six seconds—two to lift and four to lower. Jerky movements can cause injury and soreness. Fourth, stop if your muscles hurt. The dictum "No pain, no gain" is both wrong and potentially dangerous. Your muscles should feel fatigued during the last repetitions, but you should not feel sharp or piercing pains in your muscles. If you do feel pain, stop the exercise immediately. Finally, cool down after you exercise by doing a few minutes of walking or light jogging, followed by stretching again.

It is also helpful to have a well-qualified personal trainer show you proper techniques and a range of weightlifting exercises to consider. Personal trainers should have bachelor's or master's degrees in physical education or exercise physiology, and certification by the American College of Sports Medicine or the American Council on Exercise.

Excuses, Excuses

I met one of my childhood friends for dinner last year. I had not seen Tom for twenty years, and he looked good and was happy with his family life and work as a pharmacist. We talked about various things, including exercise. Tom noticed that I had lost a considerable amount of weight and seemed to be in excellent physical condition compared to the way he remembered me. He asked the usual questions about "my secret."

I discussed the importance of exercise in my life. As a health professional, he was fully aware of the value of exercising. However, he told me, "I really wish I had time for exercise." I talked about the idea of making time for exercise rather than thinking of it as an option. He argued that he "just didn't have time for it."

When I probed about this time constraint, Tom indicated that he believed exercise would interfere with his ability to earn a decent living. He wanted to work more and more hours every year to keep increasing his income. It turns out that he and his wife made a more than satisfactory income and had no major financial pressures. In fact, his wife is a successful physician and they earn more than 99% of the households in the United States. I asked, "Wouldn't you and your family be better off if you were healthier and happier, than if you made an extra few thousand dollars per year by working additional hours you could use for exercising?" Tom argued that he and his wife do not like to take out loans when they buy something like a car. I replied incredulously, "You mean that you feel a 'need' to pay for your cars in cash and that's the reason you don't exercise?" "I guess so," Tom responded weakly.

Exercise takes time and requires some sacrifice. Tom decided that the "sacrifice" of taking out a loan to buy a new car every ten years (which he and his family could easily afford) outweighed the benefits of exercising. This is a remarkable piece of rationalization.

Like most struggling weight controllers, you've probably found some creative ways to talk yourself out of exercising. What are your top ten reasons for *not* exercising? How have you argued yourself back into brisk walks in the morning or some other form of regular activity? In twenty-five years of helping people debate themselves successfully on this point, I've discovered a few of the better arguments and counterarguments. You may find reviewing some of these helpful when trying to convince yourself to take this important step in an attempt to control your weight more effectively (Table 6.4).

Preventing and Managing Injuries

Have injuries ever interfered with your exercise habits? When people injure an ankle or a back, it can take a long time, if not forever, for them to get back to regular exercising. Even minor and common illnesses, including colds, can change the momentum of consistent exercising. Exercising takes time, costs money, and interferes with your life to a significant degree. When we become sick or injured, living

TABLE 6.4 EXERCISING: EXCUSES AND RESPONSES	
EXCUSE	**RESPONSE**
I'm too tired.	Exercising will energize me. I am unwilling to give into a temporary feeling of tiredness.
I need more sleep.	It would be nice to get more sleep. Exercising will help me sleep better. I can go to sleep earlier or sleep longer tomorrow. Being a little sleepy won't hurt me.
I have more important things to do.	Making time for myself is as important as anything else. I can work more efficiently if I exercise and stay healthy. I can even think about my work while exercising to jump-start it when I get back.
I'm too busy.	What's more important to me? Exercise deserves to be a high priority in my life. It does take time. It takes time to invest in myself, my health, my well-being, my future.
I'd rather relax.	Just because I'd rather relax doesn't mean that's the best thing for me to do now. It's more important to fulfill my commitment to losing weight.
I don't feel well enough.	Unless I have a fever or I am deathly ill, I know it's safe for me to exercise. I can always exercise at a lower intensity than usual. I could walk instead of run, or I can jog slowly instead of at my usual pace. I can do at least fifteen or twenty minutes of something. I'd rather reduce my exercise than do none at all.
I'm just not motivated to do it.	I do not have to wait for some magical level of "motivation." I can "Just do it!" If I think about why I want to exercise, that will increase my motivation.
I'll do it later (or tomorrow).	If I convince myself to do it later, I might not do it at all. If I get it out of the way, I'll feel better. Every day counts. If I don't make today count, what makes me think I will make tomorrow count? My commitment is a commitment to every day. Every day counts.

without exercise becomes normal, which increases the challenge of working exercise back into a complicated life.

You have choices about managing illnesses and injuries. First, you can either expect some injuries and illnesses to interfere with your exercising, or you can just hope "It won't happen to me." The latter hope almost never works well. You can plan more effectively when your expectations fit reality better. What will you do *if* you get sick? How would you manage a back or knee injury? It helps to plan for these common problems.

Second, you can take either an aggressive or a more conservative approach to managing illnesses and injuries. The aggressive approach usually includes exercising sooner than you think you can. Doctors I've consulted often recommend resting when fevers go to one hundred degrees or more. When fevers get below one hundred degrees and you feel capable of some easy exercise, like walking, you can go for it. "Exercise a day or two before you think you can," I have heard from some very knowledgeable physicians. Consider your reaction to a doctor suggesting the more conservative (and typical), "rest until you're feeling much better." Do you simply follow that advice? You could. You could also challenge it gently by asking if you could walk for several miles or do some other low-impact workout sooner rather than later.

Consider asking your doctor specifically about the medical risks of exercising at various levels of intensity and various durations. "Can I walk three miles? Five miles? Jog slowly three miles? Use a step machine for twenty minutes? Play doubles tennis?" "Yes" or "no" answers are not good enough. Try to find out advantages and risks of various alternatives. Then decide what to do. It's your body and your commitment to weight control. If you manage it as actively as you can, you'll probably feel better about it.

You can consult your doctor about illness and exercise, but who do you consult for some of the more common exercise-related maladies? Problems with knees, backs, hips, and feet plague middle-aged exercisers as well as many highly trained twenty-year-old athletes. All athletic teams at the college level use athletic trainers to help mend these maladies quickly and avoid unnecessary damage. At Olympic events, dozens of athletic trainers help the athletes stay competitive despite various strains and sprains. You can get similar assistance at physical therapy centers. Almost all hospitals have such centers. Sometimes these centers are located in hospital rehabilitation or orthopedic clinics.

Some large-scale studies also support the effectiveness of chiropractors specifically for back problems. Sometimes foot problems lead to knee problems and/or to hip and back problems. Podiatrists can help when feet become uncooperative.

Consider investigating physical therapy, chiropractic, and podiatric alternatives. Each approach has advantages and disadvantages, depending on the nature of the problem. The key to feeling better is—you guessed it—persistence. Try to pursue various alternatives until some approach makes sense and really helps. It is frustrating. The healing arts remain more art than science, unfortunately. Support from others sometimes helps, but even without support remember the critical role exercise plays in effective weight control. You can find lower impact (or less intense) alternatives when injuries occur (walking or swimming instead of jogging or playing tennis, for example). You can refuse to stop moving whenever possible. You can manage your weight with an imperfect body. You cannot manage your weight by becoming or staying sedentary.

Safety Tips

Perhaps the best way of managing injuries is to avoid them. The American Heart Association suggests the following helpful hints:

Stretch, warm up, and cool down. Warming up for several minutes gives your body a chance to get ready for more vigorous exercise. Start at a slow to medium pace and gradually increase it for several minutes. Warm-ups can include jogging in place or just moving around slowly and beginning to orient your body to exercise. Stretching exercises are a very important part of the warm-up and should be done slowly and rhythmically. Listed below are four of the many different stretches that are widely used:

- **Wall-push.** Stand one to two feet away from a wall. Lean forward, pushing against the wall, keeping heels flat. Count to ten, then rest. Repeat one or two times.
- **Palm touch.** Stand with your feet shoulder-width apart and your knees slightly bent. Bend from the waist and try to touch your palms either to your ankles or to the floor. Do not bounce. Count to ten, then rest. Repeat this once or twice. If you have lower back problems, do this exercise with your legs crossed.
- **Toe touch.** Place your right leg on a stair, chair, or other object. Keeping your other leg straight, lean forward slowly to touch your right toe with your right hand ten times. Then do this with your left hand ten times. Again, do not bounce. Switch legs and repeat with each hand. Repeat the entire exercise one to two times.
- **Shoulder blade scratch.** Reach back with one arm as if to scratch your shoulder blade. Use the other hand to extend the stretch. Alternate arms. Repeat one to two times.

Always cool down for several minutes after exercising. The cool-down should progress slowly and gradually. For example, swim more slowly or change to a more leisurely stroke. You can also cool down by walking for several minutes after a jog. Cooling down allows your body to relax gradually. It also helps remove build-ups of the by-products of exercising that accumulate in the muscles. Abrupt stopping can cause dizziness and cramping or muscle soreness later in the day. Consider repeating your stretching and warm-up exercises to loosen up your muscles after an exercise session.

Build up your level of activity gradually. Starting out slowly helps avoid overexertion. This decreases the likelihood of injury. Remember, even if you walk at a slow pace, you accomplish much more than staying sedentary.

Listen to your body for early warning signs. You can feel pains in joints, feet, ankles, and legs quite easily when you're just getting used to exercising. Minor muscle and joint injuries can be treated readily by aspirin and rest. When you feel pain, discontinue what you are doing. If you feel a pain in your ankle when running, for example, try slowing down for a while and see if the pain goes away. If it persists, stop running. Some discomforts are perfectly normal during exercising. It may take a while for you to recognize the difference between normal discomforts and potentially problematic pains.

Be aware of possible signs of heart problems. Pain or pressure in the left or mid-chest area, left neck, shoulder, or arm during or just after exercising can be a sign of a heart problem. These sorts of pains can also occur due to the normal strains of exercising. For example, a "stitch" is a common, relatively sharp pain that occurs below the bottom of your ribs. It is a cramping of some muscles due to a temporary lack of oxygen to those muscles. Stitches stop when you slow down. Heart problems do not cause stitches. On the other hand, sudden dizziness, cold sweats, or fainting are signs of much more dangerous problems. If any of these things happen during or immediately after exercising, get medical attention right away.

Take appropriate precautions for special weather conditions. When it is hot and humid outside, consider exercising less intensely than normal for a week or so until you adapt to the heat. It also helps to exercise during cooler parts of the day such as early morning or early evening after the sun has gone down. Fluid intake becomes especially important under conditions in which you might become dehydrated (for example, when traveling or during particularly hot days). On such hot days, you might think you also need extra salt; however, you will probably get enough salt in your regular diet. Also, if you maintain a good level of physical fitness, your body learns to conserve salt and your sweat consists mostly of water.

On very hot and sunny days, the possibility of heat stroke is a concern. Signs of heat stroke include feeling dizzy, weak, light-headed, and excessively tired. Also watch for a sudden decrease in sweating and a rapid increase in body temperature. If you feel sensations very much like these, get yourself to a cooler place as soon as possible, drink some fluids, rest, and seek medical attention.

Dress appropriately for hot weather. It helps to wear very light, loose-fitting clothing. Rubberized or plastic suits, sweatshirts, and sweatpants do nothing but increase your risk of heat stroke. Such clothing does not help you lose weight any faster. It does make you sweat more, but the weight you lose in fluids by sweating is quickly replaced as soon as you begin drinking fluids again.

On cold days, wear one less layer of clothing than you would if you were outside but not exercising. Some people find that they can wear a couple of layers less than they normally would. Several layers of clothing work better than a single layer of heavier clothes. You can wear old mittens, gloves, or cotton socks to protect your hands. Some of my clients wear inexpensive cotton garden gloves while walking or running. Since up to 40% of your body's heat is lost through your neck and head, wearing a comfortable hat is especially advisable in cold weather.

Remember that rainy, icy, or snowy days make for special hazards for exercisers. Persistent weight controllers develop a variety of alternative means of exercising that allow for these weather conditions. They may use indoor tracks or machines at health clubs, play racquetball, take tennis lessons, or use their own treadmills or exercycles.

Other miscellaneous tips. Here are a few additional hints for safe exercising:

- Avoid strenuous exercise for at least two hours after eating a meal. It also aids digestion to wait about twenty minutes before eating following an exercise session.
- Proper equipment can prevent a variety of injuries. This includes good running shoes for walkers or runners and goggles to protect eyes for racquetball, handball, or squash players.
- Hard and uneven surfaces such as cement or rough fields cause

more injuries than smoother surfaces. Soft, even surfaces such as level grass fields, dirt paths, or tracks for running are better for your feet and joints.

- When you walk, run, or jog, try to land on your heels rather than on the balls of your feet. This minimizes the strain on your feet, knees, and lower legs. Try to keep your feet as close to the ground as possible without tripping. This method helps you land on your heels more so than on your toes.

- Walkers and joggers get hit by bicycles and cars more often than you might think. It helps to wear brightly colored clothes and reflective bands on clothes and shoes. Walk and jog facing the cars; this will enable drivers to notice you more and you to protect yourself more directly. The basic message is: Exercise defensively. Bicyclists can prevent injuries by wearing a helmet, using a light, and putting reflectors on their wheels for night riding. It also helps to ride in the direction of traffic and to avoid busy streets.

Many people concerned about weight have crossed the magic forty-year-old threshold into middle age. Middle-aged weight controllers commonly experience minor injuries, such as sprained ankles, painful backs, aching hips, and swollen knees. Every athlete experiences these problems as well. Remember that weight controllers are very much like athletes in training. You are attempting to push your body to a place it doesn't want to go. But your brain can take over and nudge your body forward, despite the inevitable aches and pains along the way.

Epilogue

One of my clients struggled mightily with developing a consistent exercise plan. She created the following poem during the height of her struggle:

With Wont's, You Can't

If you can't run every morning,
   then run in the evening.
If you can't run,
   then walk briskly.
If you can't walk briskly,
   just walk slowly or treadmill or bike or swim.
If you can't do any of this, let's face it,
   you "can't" because you "won't."
You can't walk,
   because you won't make it a priority.
You can succeed with some can'ts,
   but not with won'ts.
Won't you make yourself matter every day?

Step 6: Self-Monitor and Plan Consistently

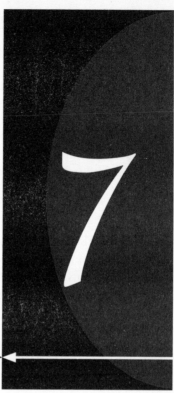

DURING OUR INITIAL INTERVIEW, Bob told me something I had heard hundreds of times before: he ate very healthfully, exercised regularly, and yet still couldn't lose the fifty extra pounds that had plagued him for twenty years. When I asked him to describe the details of his eating patterns this is what he said:

> I really do eat very healthfully. I have cereal with skim milk for breakfast typically. Sometimes I have oatmeal. I order mainly salads for lunch, with an occasional turkey sandwich. My wife cooks only very healthy foods and I don't snack very much.

When Bob actually self-monitored (observed and recorded) his eating patterns for a week, a different story emerged. It turns out Bob is the president and CEO of a fairly large information technology firm. He has more than 120 employees and they all work on the same floor. It turns out that every time an employee has a birthday, his company buys a cake for that employee. With more than 120 employees, that amounts to cakes showing up at the office several times a week. I noticed quite a few entries of "birthday cake" in Bob's food records and asked him about it. He said, "Well, I have to partake in the celebration as the boss, don't I?"

The additional dozens of extra fat grams and hundreds of calories per week seemed justified to Bob because of his role as the boss. Unfortunately, your resistant biology doesn't care whether you're the boss or not. If you eat excessive amounts of fat and calories, your body will very happily maintain your weight regardless of your general style of eating in a healthy fashion. Quite simply put:

Everything Counts!

Bob's wife Ellen also believed that she was a generally quite healthy (low-fat) eater and reported frequent exercise. She, like Bob, however, failed to lose thirty-five extra pounds despite these efforts over many years. When she and I reviewed her first week's self-monitoring records, I noticed frequent entries that looked something like: *Salad, with chicken—100 calories, 2 fat grams.* When I asked about these salads, Ellen mentioned that they did include dressing but the dressing was low in fat. I asked Ellen to describe how she knew that the dressings were low in fat and she told me the following story: "Whenever I go out to eat and order a salad I ask the server about the available dressings. At most places, the servers tell me that they have a light vinaigrette. I almost always get that light vinaigrette."

It turns out many servers describe their vinaigrette dressings as "light" as a way of distinguishing them from the heavier, creamier dressings like blue cheese and ranch. However, very rarely are these dressings actually low in calories or fat. Unless the server says "fat-free" or can show you the bottle or tell you the specific number of fat grams per tablespoon of dressing, you must assume that this is a relatively high-fat oil-based dressing. As such, a typical serving has about fifteen grams of fat and 150 or more calories in two tablespoons.

Ellen and Bob's stories simply illustrate that attending to the details is a critical element of successful weight control. In this chapter, you will read more scientific evidence about the amazing power of self-monitoring. You'll also discover a variety of ways to focus carefully on the details of your eating and exercising behaviors (i.e., self-monitoring). You'll find some that are more cumbersome and others that are very efficient. The key is to find some way for you to stay focused very consistently on these details in order to overcome your remarkably resistant biology. Finally, you'll review the top ten high-risk situations faced by serious weight controllers, and five ways to use planning and self-monitoring to manage them effectively.

The Amazing Power of Self-Monitoring

Self-monitoring is the careful observation and recording of behavior you wish to change. For weight controllers, self-monitoring involves observing and recording eating and exercising behaviors.

No weight loss expert would disagree about at least one thing: self-monitoring is the single most important aspect of effective weight control. The following list reviews several scientific studies that clearly make this point. The results demonstrate that when people write down at least 75% of their eating and exercising behaviors they often succeed in losing weight and maintaining weight loss. Writing down very little of these critical aspects of weight control usually results in very minimal or temporary success. These findings are so clear and so consistent that they support the following very dramatic assertion:

If you could maintain a written record of everything you eat and all of your exercising for the next ten years, or at least 75% of your eating and exercising behaviors, you would almost certainly become an effective weight controller.

RESEARCH FINDINGS SHOWING THE BENEFITS OF VERY CONSISTENT SELF-MONITORING:

- Among weight controllers in a twelve-week program, those who self-monitored consistently lost 64% more weight than the inconsistent self-monitors; the consistent self-monitors also maintained this superior weight loss three months later.
- Weight controllers who discontinued self-monitoring during a three-week holiday season (Thanksgiving to New Year's) gained fifty-seven times as much weight as their counterparts who continued to self-monitor consistently.

- Out of ten changes in eating habits that were measured, only self-monitoring was clearly related to successful weight loss when evaluated almost two years after the program began.
- Two studies showed that even weight controllers who generally self-monitored consistently discontinued monitoring for a day or more sometimes. During the weeks that they self-monitored inconsistently, however, they lost much less weight than was usual for them. More specifically, when these generally consistent self-monitors kept track of virtually everything they ate and all of their exercise, they lost between one and two pounds per week; during their least consistent weeks of self-monitoring they lost only 50% as much weight.
- Weight controllers who were generally inconsistent self-monitors gained an average of one pound per week during their least consistent self-monitoring weeks. They fared much better—in fact they maintained their weight—during weeks in which they self-monitored almost every day.
- Only highly consistent self-monitors lost any weight during the holiday season (Thanksgiving to New Year's) in two different studies.
- Weight controllers who self-monitored very consistently in the first few weeks of several professional treatment programs maintained much greater weight losses, compared to inconsistent self-monitors, when evaluated one to two years after treatment began.

Chart 7.1 illustrates one of the above findings.

Let's consider an example of Molly's self-monitoring records—shown below—to see how self-monitoring helped her. Before looking at her records, spend a few seconds writing down what you have eaten today thus far. Try to notice both the details of what you ate and how you felt about your eating. Also, describe your exercising and note any reactions to the process of writing all of this down.

Consider how it would have affected you, if you were Molly, to write down these foods on this particular day. Molly noted that the amount of fat she consumed on that day (thirty-five grams) exceeded her twenty gram per day goal by quite a bit. The monitoring helped her stay aware of her **goal** and to use that goal to help her change. In fact, she used her failure to meet her goal as a way of renewing her **commitment** to strive toward eating less fat the next day. Another goal Molly failed to meet concerned exercise. Molly attempts to exercise every day for at least a half-hour. She likes to swim and uses that as a primary means of exercise. On this day, she didn't fulfill that part of her mission.

CHART 7.1: SELF-MONITORING

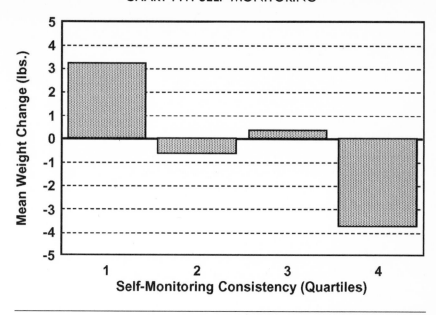

Weight controllers who self-monitored very consistently (the fourth quartile in this chart) lost much more weight than those who were less consistent (the first three quartiles). Based on research by K. Boutelle and D. Kirschenbaum published in 1998 (Further support for consistent self-monitoring as a vital component of successful weight control. *Obesity Research*, v. 6, pp. 219–224).

MOLLY'S SELF-MONITORING RECORD FOR MARCH 7

DAY/DATE: Thursday, March 7
EXERCISE: None

Time	Food	Calories	Fat Grams
7:30 A.M.	Orange juice	130	0
Noon	2 fat-free yogurts	380	0
	8 garlic breadsticks	240	8
8:00 P.M.	4 small turkey sandwiches, with Dijon mustard, (on Hawaiian buns)	600	13
	1 muffin	380	14
Total Cals./Fat Gms. =		**1,730**	**35**

Molly has noted that she feels more in **control** and generally in a more positive **mood** when she stays focused on her eating and exercising programs. Just the process of writing about and thinking about these important aspects of her life makes her feel better about herself. She also uses self-monitoring to stay aware of certain **eating patterns** and to focus on the **details** of what she eats and under what circumstances. She has learned that in order to achieve success in weight control "the devil is in the details."

On this particular day, she realized that she neglected to eat any fruit or vegetables. Eating such excellent forms of fiber help keep her digestion moving along effectively and also decrease the risk of colon cancer. This is one of her weaknesses and something she consistently tries to change. The details of her eating also showed relatively minimal consumption of protein from the time she woke up until eight P.M. This lack of protein, lack of fruits and vegetables, and substitution primarily of carbohydrates and sweets (albeit fat-free sweets) could certainly increase the chance of eating in a less-controlled way in the evening. For example, she rarely eats muffins with 380 calories and fourteen grams of fat. Yet, on this day, with its imbalanced plan earlier in the day, she wound up consuming the vast majority of her fat grams after eight P.M. On a more positive note, she chose turkey for her sandwich meat and clearly limited her total intake to a very modest amount—until the evening.

The following points summarize the benefits of self-monitoring Molly realized and that you could experience by self-monitoring consistently. The most important of these can help you persist in efforts over time despite the inevitable frustrations. Increasing your commitment and committing to focusing on the details can keep you going when the scale doesn't cooperate or after you eat some high-fat foods. Remember: The devil is in the details!

WHY SELF-MONITORING HELPS

Consistent self-monitoring improves weight control by:

- Increasing ability to use GOALS
- Improving COMMITMENT to change
- Increasing feelings of CONTROL
- Improving understanding of EATING/EXERCISE PATTERNS
- Improving information about, and focus on, the DETAILS
- Promoting more POSITIVE MOODS

Self-Monitoring Techniques

Self-Monitoring: A Good Idea in 1500 and Today

Some really good ideas have no time limit. In the sixteenth century, St. Ignatius Loyola suggested that self-monitoring can help people improve their lives. He suggested self-monitoring twice a day, every day:

> [A person who wishes to change himself] should demand an account of himself with regard to the particular point which he has resolved to watch in order to correct himself and improve. Let him go over the single hours or periods from the time he arose to the hour and moment of the present examination and make a mark for each time he has fallen into the particular sin or defect.
>
> The second day should be compared with the first, that is, the two examinations of the present day with the two of the preceding day. Let him observe if there is an improvement from one day to another. Let him compare one week with another and observe whether he has improved during the present week as compared to the preceding.

Present-day weight controllers have choices among dozens of different methods of recording information about their eating and exercising behaviors. Every bookstore sells various weight loss diaries. Some weight controllers use laptops, PDAs, dictation, and calendars to self-monitor. Science cannot tell you which particular format will help you self-monitor. Based on more than thirty years of experience helping thousands of weight controllers, I have seen many successful weight controllers use three variations of self-monitoring techniques very effectively: basic self-monitoring, condensed self-monitoring, and computerized self-monitoring.

The passages below give examples of each of these approaches. By reviewing them carefully, you can find a technique that you can use most comfortably and consistently. Remember, consistency in self-monitoring is the key. Whatever technique you use, in order for you to succeed at losing weight, you have to find an approach that you are very likely to use every single day. After achieving your weight loss goal and maintaining it for many months, you can decrease your self-monitoring. At that point, you can simply weigh yourself on a regular basis (at least weekly) and then use self-monitoring if your weight begins to increase by a couple of pounds. In this way, self-monitoring is a tool that you can use throughout your life to increase your ability to focus very specifically on your eating and exercising patterns. No matter what self-monitoring technique you use or how long you need to keep it up, accuracy is the key, as the box below illustrates.

IS THAT AN APPLE YOU'RE EATING—OR A SMALL WATERMELON?

Does an apple = an apple = an apple? Very consistent self-monitoring, even if inaccurate, greatly improves effectiveness at weight control. But consistent and accurate self-monitoring is even more useful and effective. To achieve accurate self-monitoring, it helps to know the details of the size of typical portions. Try taking the quiz below and see how accurately you can judge some common portion sizes:

Question 1. A medium-sized orange or apple is about the same size as:
  A. A small basketball
  B. A tennis ball
  C. A grapefruit

Question 2. A three-ounce portion of meat is about the same size as:
  A. An iPod
  B. Your head
  C. A deck of cards

Question 3. A one-ounce portion of cheese is about the size of:
  A. A deck of cards
  B. A 3.5-inch computer disk
  C. A VW Beetle

Question 4. A teaspoon of margarine is about the same size as:
  A. A CD
  B. Your nose
  C. The tip of your thumb

Answers: 1–B; 2–A&C; 3–B; 4–C

Basic Self-Monitoring

Jan's story below shows an example of her use of the basic self-monitoring technique. By far the most important aspect of basic self-monitoring is the recording of specific information about all foods eaten every day. Whether or not you record details, such as calories consumed and fat grams consumed, is far less important than the recording of your food intake and your exercise efforts. On the other hand, recording and totaling calories and fat grams consumed allows you to use the power of goal-setting to your advantage.

JAN'S FINAL BATTLE

Jan was a forty-two-year-old public relations executive when she began what she called her "final battle." Jan had many issues concerning food that resulted in anorexia (extreme thinness due to self-starvation) as a young adult, followed by a substantial weight problem for most of her life. At the time she began her last vigorous effort to lose weight, she stood five feet four inches tall and weighed 242 pounds.

Jan noted that the weight problem (approximately one hundred pounds overweight) bothered her tremendously every single day of her life. Yet, after trying everything that she could think of to beat it, she had given up on it in the past couple of years. That only made it worse. She was disgusted with the way she looked. Jan had enjoyed clothes very much and was a very good-looking woman. She felt that this excess weight had tremendously undermined her life at work, her relationship with her husband (primarily due to her own unhappiness more than anything else), and her physical well-being. Jan was very knowledgeable about nutrition, having studied it in college. She was just determined to find some way to win this final battle.

By self-monitoring very carefully, attending weekly individual therapy sessions with me, and religiously and consistently developing a treadmill/walking exercise program, Jan became very successful at weight control. She used her considerable knowledge about food and cooking to create a wide variety of interesting soups and other concoctions. Her husband was fully supportive of her efforts and actually enjoyed the change in patterns and types of foods at home. After approximately eleven months of hard work on this aspect of her life, Jan got below the two-hundred-pound barrier. Continued efforts in the following six months brought her weight down to a much more

comfortable 172 pounds. Over the past two years her weight has fluc-
tuated between 160 and 175 pounds. Although she would like to get
below 150, she found that even at 170 pounds she is able to wear very
attractive clothes and has dramatically improved her self-esteem and
physical well-being.

Jan exercises almost every day, often walking as much as five miles
at a time on a treadmill or on Chicago's lakefront. Jan's blood pressure
has decreased, her cholesterol is lower, and she is much stronger than
she has been in many years. She feels good and is in a much better
mood almost every day compared to how she felt several years ago.
She believes she generally lives a more balanced life now.

Jan still struggles, however, to stay pleased and grateful (largely to
herself) for what she has achieved. She focuses, at least sometimes, in
a mean-spirited way, on the unfinished business of those last twenty
pounds. Perhaps this edge of staying only partially satisfied with her
weight control efforts has helped her maintain the seventy-pound
weight loss for two years:

> I've never maintained my weight—not even for a month! When I think
> of that, I feel very good to look and feel and be 170 pounds instead of
> 240 pounds. I've got to stay positive about what I've done, but avoid eas-
> ing up on my approach to food or exercise. I know there's a 240-pound-
> er in me, lurking, waiting for me to give in to extra sleep, snack on real
> potato chips, or say "What the hell!" in other ways. My self-monitoring
> is my insurance policy: It fends off that hungry 240-pounder.

Below is an example of a typical day of Jan's basic self-monitoring:

JAN'S SELF-MONITORING RECORD

DAY/DATE: Friday, March 12
EXERCISE: 3.5 miles (treadmill)

Time	Food	Calories	Fat Grams
Noon	2-ounce sourdough roll	200	2
	Steamed carrots	50	0
	3 steamed red potatoes	200	0
	6 ounces broiled swordfish	300	9
7:00 P.M.	1½ cups brown rice	300	0
	Small baked potato	100	0

	2 teaspoons fat-free		
	sour cream	30	0
	1 chicken breast	170	4
	2 teaspoons hot and		
	sour sauce	30	0
	Steamed veggies	50	0
10:00 P.M.	Orange	100	0
	½ cup fat-free yogurt	100	0
Total Cals./Fat Gms. =		**1,630**	**15**

Jan used the goal of twenty fat grams per day so that she could make adjustments in the evening if necessary to reach that goal every day. Certainly on some days, Jan did not record the amount of fat grams consumed. Here's the way she compared the difference between recording and totaling fat grams versus just recording and totaling food consumed:

Whenever I total the amount of fat grams I eat, I become much more tuned in to the little details that squeak in around the edges in my eating program. For example, at a party it's very easy to eat a little cube of cheese on a cracker. If you don't record the fat grams, which could quite easily be five for small cubes of cheese, I found I could talk myself into thinking it wasn't much of anything. When I get oriented to counting and focusing on every single fat gram, that's when I eliminate the cheese from that cracker and that's when I lose more weight.

It also helps to record the total amount eaten in calories, as well the total number of fat grams consumed. Without recording calories, you'll tend to "forget" the actual amounts of food you ate. On the other hand, people have the greatest difficulties when they discontinue self-monitoring altogether or only record some of what they eat during the day. One way of thinking about this is that perhaps 80% of the benefit from self-monitoring is gained from recording eating and exercising in a consistent fashion. You can gain another 20% of the benefits of self-monitoring by recording calories and fat consumed.

Some self-monitoring formats require just too much work, unless you are a particularly obsessive individual. Some of the available self-monitoring books ask you to record how you are feeling, situations that you found yourself in and do other fairly elaborate things associated with your eating and exercising patterns. Research generally supports the following acronym: KISS (Keep It Simple, Silly). The most important aspect of self-monitoring is to stay focused every day. The focusing decreases tremendously if you overburden yourself with writing out largely unnecessary details.

Condensed Self-Monitoring

Most people get the appropriate level of information and keep themselves from being overburdened by using basic self-monitoring. However, what if you reach a reasonable weight and have been self-monitoring for years? At that point, you just might benefit from a device that helps you stay a bit more aware and focused than otherwise. That is the best rationale for using condensed self-monitoring. Condensed self-monitoring provides a very quick method to keep you focused on total calories consumed per day, total fat grams consumed, and amount and consistency of exercising.

Take a look at Cindy's story and see if you can understand why she—having lost 263 pounds and maintaining that loss for more than five years—chose to use condensed self-monitoring. As shown in Cindy's story below, Cindy found it quite useful to write down simply the number of calories she consumed every day and her exercise. This type of self-monitoring takes only a few seconds per day, yet the payoff can be much better maintenance of weight loss.

Research on setting goals in business contexts shows that setting specific challenging goals improves performance by 16%, on average. In weight control, that might translate to someone who typically eats 1,500 calories per day managing to eat 1,260 calories per day. It also translates into exercising for thirty-five minutes per day instead of thirty minutes per day. These differences may not seem like much, but they add up. They can mean the difference between maintaining weight for a year versus gaining several pounds per year.

THE KEY TO CINDY'S HUGE SUCCESS:
CLEAR FOCUSING AND CONTROLLED BINGE-EATING

Cindy lost 263 pounds! She began this journey at five feet two inches and 403 pounds. Four years later she weighed 140 pounds. Cindy reported that she had "given up" on many aspects of her life when she was so heavy. She just barely managed to go to work and survive. At this new healthy weight, she has experienced a major rebirth in her interests in music, other people, and herself.

Cindy believes some of the keys to her remarkable success include exercising every day (brisk walk for forty-five minutes), weather permitting. The only weather that doesn't permit such activity, according to Cindy, is a wind chill that is twenty-five degrees below zero or even colder. Since that only happens a few times a year in Chicago, Cindy can be found walking in her neighborhood virtually every day before going to work.

Another critical aspect that helped Cindy lose the equivalent of two other people in weight is her new method of binge-eating. Cindy has always had difficulties with binges. When she feels stressed or bored, for as long as she can remember, she has often eaten large quantities of food. When she weighed four hundred pounds, those foods included milkshakes, French fries, cookies, and other high-fat items. Now, a binge might include ten cups of air-popped popcorn and three pears. She believes in the idea: *Deviate Quantitatively, Not Qualitatively*. In other words, Cindy knows that she can eat fairly large quantities of very low-fat foods without compromising her weight control efforts. On the other hand, deviations that include eating some high-fat foods can cause rather immediate and dramatic weight gains. This occurs in part because once that barrier is broken, the tendency to eat more and other types of high-fat foods increases. Remember the potato chip company ad that said, "Bet you can't eat just one?" They were right.

Cindy has maintained her focus for many years by using a condensed form of self-monitoring. She has a little book where she writes down the number of calories consumed during the course of the day. For example:

Day/Date: Tuesday, April 1
Exercise: 45 minutes walking
Calories Consumed:

150

250

200

350

200

75

50

1,275

These are some of Cindy's comments about her method of staying focused:

I'm not sure what it is about this approach to self-monitoring that works, but it does—at least for me. I aim for 1,200 calories every day. By writing down these numbers I can see how close I'm getting. It helps me stay alert about quantities. I eat so little fat anyway that I don't find it necessary to keep track of that. So, I'm mainly interested in the numbers of calories and trying to beat my goal every day.

Some days I realize that I've gone over a reasonable amount by the end of lunch. By looking at these numbers, I can make a mid-day correction and eat a particularly light dinner.

It's so easy to "forget" things you eat—especially when you wish you hadn't eaten them. I think this condensed self-monitoring keeps the details real and helps me feel in control.

You can see another variation on condensed self-monitoring by reviewing Ann's story below. Ann found she was able to maintain her focus and her weight when she wrote down numbers of calories consumed in her appointment book. A somewhat technical explanation for the benefits Ann appreciated about her approach to self-monitoring concerns the premack principle, already discussed on page 64, which asserts that you can increase desirable behaviors by pairing those behaviors with events that occur frequently. In Ann's approach to condensed self-monitoring, she paired the frequent event, looking at her appointment book (something that she did at least five times per day), with a desirable behavior that she wanted to increase (focusing on her weight control effort).

ANN'S BREATHER

Ann was in her late thirties when we first met. She was pregnant and very concerned about eating and her weight problem. She was five feet tall and weighed 198 pounds. The pregnancy was only in its tenth week, so Ann's weight was stable—but approximately seventy pounds over where she would have liked it to be.

Ann struggled with weight most of her adult life. She was constantly trying out various diets. She had her second child three years before seeing me for the first time, and had been gaining weight rather steadily and at what she considered to be an alarming rate. She had never been at this weight and found it extremely distressing. She prided herself on her looks, enjoyed lots of interesting clothes when she was slimmer, and wanted to get back to a place where she could feel good about herself and the way she looked. Ann was in a business that involved many meetings with business groups. She simply felt much more unsure about herself with this increased weight gain. She also found it increasingly difficult to keep up with her active young children. In addition, she wanted to feel good and be as healthy as she could during the pregnancy.

Ann began self-monitoring using the basic approach. She also focused on attempting to use her treadmill at least thirty minutes per day. Ann radically reduced the amount of fat she consumed (from approximately eighty fat grams per day, down to fifteen fat grams per day). Ann's weight stabilized with this approach, despite the growing fetus within her.

After Ann's baby was born, she lost weight steadily over the next six months and got to a much healthier and more comfortable weight of 148 pounds. Her exercise was fairly consistent, she ate between 800 and 1,200 calories per day, and ate very little fat. She kept her self-monitoring booklet religiously, only missing a few days during the entire twenty-six weeks it took her to lose forty pounds. Ann still struggled with the exercise aspect periodically. She found it difficult to exercise in the morning and then got home from work feeling exhausted and wanting to spend time with her children. Fortunately, she had a very supportive husband who encouraged her and provided her with the leeway to exercise in the evenings on most days.

Ann's weight loss came to a somewhat surprising halt after the initial forty pounds. It turns out that she was undergoing a variety of fertility enhancement procedures. This focus and renewed energy spent on becoming pregnant again decreased her interest in weight control. At the heart of it was her view that if she became pregnant (or when she became pregnant) she would no longer be able to continue losing weight anyway. It was simply too difficult for her to focus very vigorously on losing weight when she knew that biologically the effort would be modified considerably sometime relatively soon (she hoped).

She and I decided to meet less frequently and to alter her self-monitoring technique in accord with her desire to take a "breather" from a truly intensely focused effort at losing weight. The plan for the breather was to continue the same style of eating that had gotten her to this new and much happier state. The goal was also to maintain exercise for similar reasons. In order to increase the likelihood that that would occur, Ann decided to keep track of the calories she consumed per day in her appointment book. This process only took a few seconds, but those were a few seconds used wisely. When she wrote down what she was eating, she thought about it. She thought about whether it was meeting her standards in terms of fat consumption and total calories. She thought about her goal of eating approximately 1,100 to 1,300 calories per day. She thought about why this mattered in the long run. Ann considered the fact that she had made major strides in the past four months and that she didn't want to throw that away. She also realized that if she wasn't focused when she became pregnant, it might get very easy to gain excessive amounts of weight.

Ann found that by writing down numbers of calories consumed in her appointment book, she realized that she was eating less fruit and fewer vegetables than she had been in the past. This information helped her modify her eating patterns to decrease her appetite and improve her digestive system.

Monday, March 8 Calories

Time	Event	Calories
7:00		250
8:00		
9:00		
10:00	Staff Meeting	100
11:00		
12:00	Lunch with Joan	350
1:00		
2:00		
3:00	Charlie	
4:00		150
5:00	Michael	
6:00	Call Alice	
7:00		
8:00		450
		1,300

Condensed self-monitoring probably helped Ann maintain her weight because she not only recorded the number of calories she consumed in her appointment book, but she taught herself to analyze where the calories were coming from. She also considered why it was a good thing to stay focused and how she could make each day an effective day. If Ann just blindly wrote down a bunch of numbers, that would do her no good. She had to learn how to attach some meaning to those numbers to re-awaken her commitment to weight control.

Computerized Self-Monitoring

In the age of laptops, smart phones that have an app for everything, instant messaging and texting, and related technological developments, computerized self-monitoring has become increasingly popular with my clients. Arlene's and Karl's stories below show two examples of computerized self-monitoring. In the first, Arlene found it motivating to record her eating and exercising within her e-mail account at home, but also to send a copy of it to her e-mail account at work. By corresponding with herself in this way, she kept herself thinking about the importance of her weight control effort.

ARLENE: YOU'VE GOT E-MAIL—FROM YOURSELF!

Arlene, a forty-one-year-old stockbroker and mother of two, began this most recent weight control effort at five feet six inches and 210 pounds. Arlene came from a tradition of relatively high-fat eating and had never followed a consistent exercise regimen. She began self-monitoring and using a basic technique (writing in a small pocket-sized book). Her exercise approach emphasized everyday activities, such as walking to and from a train to get to work, as opposed to a more formal and consistent routine every morning. That was one of her weaknesses as a weight controller. In addition, her history of high-fat eating was difficult to leave completely behind, which was required for this intensive method of weight control. After some major changes in her job and her husband's job, she found herself regaining some of the sixty pounds that she had lost over the past two years.

When Arlene's weight started approaching two hundred pounds again, she decided she had to find a way to self-monitor that could help her maintain her interest. Being very familiar with computers, she created a self-monitoring technique utilizing her two e-mail accounts. At the end of every day she e-mailed her records to her work e-mail address. As soon as she got to work she was reminded by her computer: "You've got mail!" This forced her to take a look at her records on a regular basis. She just kept sending messages back and forth to herself about her eating and exercising patterns.

The initial enthusiasm for this new e-mail self-monitoring technique helped Arlene re-lose about ten pounds. Some vacationing interrupted this approach, however. That's one of its disadvantages. Many people do not want to take their laptops with them when they go on vacations or travel. Arlene had become somewhat dependent on this vehicle as a means for self-monitoring. Of course, she could have always resorted to a basic self-monitoring approach while traveling. But, being a mere mortal, she didn't do that. She regained some of the initial ten pounds that she had lost. But, once her normal routine returned, so did her e-mail self-monitoring. Arlene got her weight to the low 170s again after a few additional months of hard labor.

DAY/DATE: Tuesday, October 20
EXERCISE: 20 min. gym + walking to and from the train + 8 blks. walk
WEIGHT: 171 lbs.

Time	Food	Calories	Fat Grams
6:30 A.M.	Milk in coffee	20	0
	2 saltines w/ham	60	0.5
7:30 A.M.	Milk in coffee	20	0
1:00 P.M.	Veggie burrito	30	5
	Instant soup	80	3.5
5:00 P.M.	FF Olestra chips	75	0
6:00 P.M.	Strawberry FF shake	70	0
7:00 P.M.	Slice of bread	70	1
8:00 P.M.	Stuffed egg white w/FF sour cream + mustard	50	0
	Broiled swordfish	260	8.8
	Boiled ½ potato	80	0
	Skim milk latte	50	0
11:00 P.M.	Boiled egg white	20	0
Total Cals./Fat Gms. =		**885**	**18.8**

Karl's story shows a more traditional use of the computer. Karl is a computer specialist (software consultant). He has a computer with him at almost all times and finds it very easy to use existing software programs to analyze his self-monitoring data. Nutritional software programs automatically total calories and fat eaten by the end of each day and summarize this information at the end of each week. Many of these programs also provide color graphics to show patterns over days, weeks, and months. The disadvantage of this approach is that it requires fluency with typing, tolerance for some missing information in the software programs, and a willingness to put some extra time into self-monitoring.

KARL'S SELF-MONITORING VIA SOFTWARE

Karl's 402 pounds began taking a very major toll on his life and well-being, even at the relatively young age of thirty-four.

His five-foot-ten-inch frame simply couldn't support that amount of weight. He began a series of hospitalizations because of problems maintaining circulation in his legs. He also started experiencing increasing difficulties walking and keeping up with his two young children. Karl maintained his own small computer software consultation business, and his health problems began interfering with his vitality and his eagerness to develop the business to its full potential.

Karl used his substantial skills with computers and software to self-monitor. Through consistent self-monitoring, major changes in the fat content of his eating, and the beginnings of a walking exercise program, Karl lost nearly seventy-five pounds in just six months. At the time of this writing, he has shown no signs of decelerating these efforts.

One of the things Karl noticed through his very diligent and complete self-monitoring was that in the weeks his daily fat intake averaged above twenty fat grams, his rate of weight loss declined considerably. In contrast, when his fat consumption averaged closer to ten grams per day, his rate of weight loss seemed to double. Take a look at the following two examples of Karl's self-monitoring data generated on a software program. The first example certainly shows relatively low-fat eating; but the second example shows the more extreme low-fat eating advocated in this book. The latter style of eating was the one associated with more dramatic weight loss.

A SOMEWHAT HIGHER FAT INTAKE DAY

DAY/DATE: February 11
EXERCISE: 25 min. swinging golf clubs; 25 min. walk
WEIGHT: 171 lbs.

Food	Calories	Fat Grams
1 muffin, no fat	150.00	0.00
1 cup milk, no fat	90.00	0.00
2 cups milk, no fat	180.00	0.00
2 hotdogs, no fat, BallPark	90.00	0.00
2 slices bread, wheat	130.00	2.05

Food	Calories	Fat Grams
1 chips, Wow	75.00	0.00
1 cookies, no fat, oatmeal raisin	100.00	0.00
½ cup beans, green, ButterSce, GrnGiant	30.00	1.00
½ cup rice & sauce, LngGrn/Wild, Liptn	121.30	0.20
½ chicken breast, no skin, roasted	85.80	1.86
1 chicken thigh, no skin, roasted	64.79	3.37
1 chicken wing, w/skin, roasted	60.90	4.09
1 chicken leg, w/skin, roasted	160.10	9.29
2 cups milk, no fat	180.00	0.00
1 cake, carrot, Wt. Watchers	170.0	5.00
2 cups milk, no fat	180.00	0.00
½ cup ice cream, fat-free, chc/vn	100.00	0.00
Total Cals./Fat Gms. =	**1,967.89**	**26.86**

A LOW-FAT INTAKE DAY

Day/Date: February 17
Exercise: 4x15 min. walks, bowling

Food	Calories	Fat Grams
1 muffin, no fat	150.00	0.00
1 cup milk, no fat	90.00	0.00
2 slices bread, wheat	130.00	2.05
2 ounces turkey, breast, slices, Louis Rich	81.00	1.42
1 cup lettuce, iceberg, raw	2.60	0.04
1 tomato, red, ripe, raw	25.83	0.41
1 small bag chips, baked, Frito Lay	130.00	1.50
3 cups milk, no fat	270.00	0.00
3 slices bread, wheat	195.00	3.07
2 hotdogs, no fat, BallPark	90.00	0.00
3 ounces bologna, fat-free, Oscar M	210.00	0.00
1 small bag Doritos, Wow	90.00	1.00
8 fluid ounces soup, chicken broth, no fat	39.04	0.00
¼ chicken breast, no skin, stewed	21.52	0.43
.25 mushrooms, boiled	0.81	0.01
⅓ ounce pasta, fresh, cooked	11.14	0.09
1 tablespoon onion, boiled	6.60	0.03
.30 garlic, raw	1.34	0.00

½ cup ice cream, fat-free, chc/vn	100.00	0.00
1 cup milk, no fat	90.00	0.00
Total Cals./Fat Gms. =	**1,734.88**	**10.05**

Conclusions about Self-Monitoring

Every diet encourages you to decrease your eating and change the type of eating that you do. Diets also attempt to give you hope, help you focus on this issue in your life, and, perhaps most importantly, help you increase your awareness of eating and exercising. The helpful aspects of any diet lie in these factors, not in the magic of grapefruit or the latest ideas in combining foods. The scientific approach I advocate cuts directly to the chase and provides a method of staying very clearly aware of your eating and exercising patterns every day and every week. This awareness tells you the single most important concept in self-monitoring:

Everything Counts!

Weight control does not begin on a Monday or on the first day of a new month or on the first day of a new year. It begins as soon as you can stay focused and make a sincere effort to control your eating and exercising. By self-monitoring very consistently, you learn that even if you start the day with bacon and eggs, you can finish the day with low-fat eating. Bacon and eggs do not contain an infinite number of calories or fat grams. You can count the fat grams in any food and realize that you can neutralize the effects of whatever problem food you consumed by eating more effectively at your next opportunity. Self-monitoring can help you do that. *If you cannot live with the notion that everything counts, you will not succeed at weight control.*

Self-monitoring can take many forms. Regardless of the form it takes, it must include some written record of your eating and exercising that covers every day. It should also include a record of your weight. If you know how much you are eating and exercising and know your weight at any given point in time, you are staying in the struggle to succeed. If you give up this knowledge, you allow your biology to take over. Whether you monitor via computer or use some condensed version of self-monitoring, *you can find a way to succeed if you can find a way to stay aware of the details.*

Using Self-Monitoring
and Planning to Master High-Risk Situations

Weight control does not occur in a vacuum. The young campers from Wellspring Camps that you read about in Chapter 1 and the students from the Academy of the Sierras live in environments that are perfectly tailored to support all aspects of successful weight control. The chart you saw in that chapter showed that their results were about eight to ten times better than those participating in a professional program in a clinic or hospital. Much of the difference between campers and boarding school students versus those who live in the real world occurs because of the many high-risk situations faced by weight controllers when negotiating their everyday lives. Let's consider ten of the most difficult of those situations and review how self-monitoring and planning can help you negotiate them masterfully:

10. **Coffee breaks.** Coffee breaks and other breaks in your usual routine create challenges for a variety of reasons. First, drinking coffee and other beverages has become associated with eating for most people. If you wander into a coffee shop, like Starbucks, you see many high-fat tempting bakery items close to eye view as you order your coffee. It's one thing to have a coffee with skim milk as a break. That is a pleasant treat that can fill you up and also provide a bit of protein from the skim milk. However, the very second you order a piece of carrot cake or a cheese Danish or a scone to accompany your skim milk and coffee drink, you create a world of trouble.

Take a look at the following nutritional information about some favorite coffee break add-ons:

- Starbuck's Butterscotch Scone: 520 calories, 27 fat grams
- Starbuck's Iced Carrot Cake: 540 calories, 13 fat grams
- Dunkin Donut's Glazed Donut: 240 calories, 15 fat grams
- Starbuck's Coffee Cake: 360 calories, 18 fat grams
- Au Bon Pain Plain Bagel: 370 calories, 2 fat grams

Coffee breaks in an office setting can also become associated with chips or dips or some other problematic foods. In addition, some of the more creative modern coffee drinks go well beyond a cup of coffee, more into the realm of dessert. Consider the following offerings from our friends at Starbucks once again:

- Chocolate Brownie Frappuccino, Grande: 370 calories, 9 fat grams
- Hot chocolate, Grande: 340 calories, 15 fat grams
- Carmel Macchiato, Grande: 320 calories, 14 fat grams
- Café Latte with whole milk, Grande: 260 calories, 14 fat grams

9. **When you feel stressed, pressured, anxious, or frustrated.** Try asking a few of your friends who have never had a weight problem what happens to their eating when they feel stressed. You'll find very consistently that never-overweight people eat less when upset, whereas overweight and formerly overweight people eat more. Some people argue that this is one of the reasons overweight people gain more weight during holidays than they do during non-holiday times. There is the pressure and intensity of holiday periods, colored sometimes by family issues and conflicts and omnipresent high-fat foods. In addition, feelings of frustration tend to accompany long-term problems or tasks. Working on difficult projects and trying to accomplish something that has frustration built into it often decreases free time and sleep. Sleep deprivation, in turn, leads to a lessening of restraint and greater amounts of eating. These emotions can also decrease exercising and activity. Decreases in those arenas can lead to weight gain in addition to increases in hunger.

8. **Food cravings.** Have you heard or felt any of the following:
"Sometimes I just feel like having a steak."
"I had this huge uncontrollable urge for chocolate."

In the earlier chapter on biological forces (Chapter 3: *Know the Enemy—Your Biology*), you became aware that you must struggle against a biology that wants you to eat and gain weight. This biological pressure toward eating sometimes emerges in the form of a craving. A craving is no more or less than a strong biological feeling of wanting food accompanied by a specific image of a certain type of food. To put that in the form of an equation: Food Cravings = Biological Urge to Eat + Image of a Specific Food.

7. **Business meetings where food and drink are abundant.** The classic business conference in which muffins and other pastries are being eaten by almost everyone creates a strong urge to eat such problem foods. Other business meetings can include cocktail hours with

high-fat hors d'oeuvres. Drinking alcohol decreases restraint and such decreases accompanied by the presence of high-fat food often lead to difficulties.

6. **Arriving home from work or school, tired, bored, alone.** This is the time when most people are at their hungriest. It's been a while since lunch, it's nearing dinnertime, and there is that gap of time to fill before dinner. Many of my clients have told me about standing in their kitchens eating large quantities of pretzels, potato chips, and variations on ice cream or frozen yogurt before they even put down their coats or work materials. In addition to feeling substantial hunger, the tranquilizing properties of eating become extremely appealing at a time like that.

5. **Holidays (especially Halloween, Thanksgiving, Christmas, Hanukkah).** Each holiday presents its special challenges. For example, Halloween can include excessive amounts of little chocolate treats. These candies pack a huge wallop in terms of fat grams and calories. Their diminutive size makes many weight controllers think that they have little impact. However, consider the fact that each chocolate Hershey's Kiss has 2.5 fat grams. Mini candy bars often have five or six fat grams each. When eating a few thinking that they don't amount to much, weight controllers suddenly can exceed a daily allotment of twenty fat grams—and usually well beyond that—in just a few bites. Also, the high-sugar content increases appetite, as does the high-fat content. The other holidays often involve large feasts surrounded by family members and sometimes by family conflict. This overabundance of high-fat food, in addition to the tension sometimes created by these events at this time of year, can lead to excessive eating. Even leftovers from these feasts present their own challenge.

4. **Small dinner parties.** One of the most helpful things about holidays for weight controllers is their predictability. Thanksgiving, for example, is an elaborate turkey dinner. Many families also have traditions at these holiday meals that can be visualized and predicted with considerable accuracy. This affords a better opportunity for planning and constructing a useful scenario that would allow you to get through such events unscathed. In contrast, small dinner parties thrown by friends often include surprises. These surprises include types of food served, amounts of food, limitations in choices, and sometimes considerable pressure from the host to eat certain problematic items. At smaller parties such as these, it becomes more difficult to minimize your eating without getting undesirable attention.

3. **Big parties.** Bigger parties often involve drinking or other rec-

reational drug use that can decrease inhibitions. They typically also include considerable high-fat foods and some tensions about meeting and talking to people. In addition, at big parties you are surrounded by people who are overeating and drinking too much, quite possibly prompting similar behaviors from you. For small parties, you may be able to call the host and influence the type of food served or the choices available. For bigger parties, usually most people don't make such requests and wrongly assume that enough options will appear to allow you to stay on your program.

2. **Restaurants: Business occasions.** Eating at restaurants creates problems based on type of food served and food preparation. In business situations, most people feel less comfortable making fairly elaborate special requests from the server if that becomes necessary. Some people also feel a certain pressure to eat in a manner similar to colleagues or clients in order to keep them comfortable and minimize unwanted attention. Most restaurants also serve rather large portions and encourage consumption of things like dessert.

1. **Restaurants: Recreational occasions.** All of the problems for the previous item pertaining to restaurants, such as the large portion sizes and encouragement to eat problematic foods, also occur in recreational settings when going to restaurants with friends and family. This more relaxed atmosphere may encourage you to modify elements of the menu to suit your program. This type of eating tops the list of high-risk situations because it occurs very frequently in our culture, increasingly so over the last few decades. On average, we are consuming about a third or more of our calories outside of the home. Most of these meals occur at restaurants in relatively relaxed settings with friends and families.

Five Strategies for Managing High-Risk Situations Successfully

The high-risk situations you face by themselves won't determine your success. The manner in which you handle those situations, however, will make all the difference. Please review the following strategies and see which ones you implement regularly, which ones you could develop further in your repertoire, and how you will stay committed to using these strategies when confronted with challenges:

- *Eating.* High-risk situations generally involve eating. Fortunately, you can make effective choices about what you eat in these circumstances. For example, most restaurants include grilled chicken, vegetables, low-fat soups, salads, and related items that work just fine for your eating plan. In addition, when emotions bubble up that have produced problematic eating in the past, you can now replace that style of eating with consuming higher quantities of good-quality food for your program. You'll recall that my clients have eaten fairly large quantities of such things as fruit, low-fat popcorn, and even frozen yogurt under challenging circumstances. They did this by remembering one of the key points in the *Wellspring Plan*:

Deviate quantitatively, not qualitatively.

You may also recall the excellent results obtained at the Wellspring Camps and at the boarding school (the Academy of the Sierras) that I've been helping to develop. These programs include "uncontrolled foods" at every meal. Such foods are not controlled by the staff; the students decide how much of them to eat at every meal. They include low-density foods like soups, salads, and fruits. This may be the first example of institutionalizing the principle of deviating quantitatively, not qualitatively. Such an approach produces excellent outcomes and is supported by considerable research showing the advantages of eating large quantities of low-density foods, particularly when stressed.

• *Drinking.* One of my most successful clients would routinely drink wine spritzers (wine diluted with soda water or seltzer) when attending parties. Drinking nonalcoholic or low alcohol content beverages can help decrease hunger and give you an alternative focus at such events. Liquids expand your stomach, which decreases at least one of the major signals of hunger (stomach volume) and quite possibly decreases some hormonal responses that produce hunger (ghrelin, for example).

Another drinking-related strategy involves the placement of the drink in your hand. Consider placing a drink in your dominant hand (right hand for righties). This may keep you from reaching for food and uses a principle known as "chaining." The chaining principle means that if you can increase the steps or links in your chain of behaviors from the urge to eat to the time you actually eat, you will improve your ability to control problematic eating.

- *Moving: Activity decreases appetite.* When you move, your body responds by producing hormones that decrease appetite. This is part of the "fight or flight" syndrome. This syndrome was particularly useful to our ancestors when confronted by predators. It enables the body to redirect energy from digestion and other normal processes and put that energy into your muscles, allowing you to run faster and further. Even slow or modest movements produce some of these effects and you can use them to your advantage.

  One of the best ways to start a holiday is to go for a walk or exercise in some way. That activity level at the beginning of the day does many positive things for you. It increases your sense of commitment and activates your body in an effective manner. It also redirects your attention at the very beginning of the day. You will now focus more on taking good care of yourself and less on problematic foods or conflicts that detract from your *Wellspring Plan*.

  Even moving around during dinner parties can produce desirable effects. For example, when servers come to present desserts to your fellow diners, you can get up from the table and take a restroom break or just walk around a little bit and get some fresh air. Then you can return while these particularly problematic and possibly tempting foods have been consumed or at least partially consumed. This increases your ability to focus and remember what you are trying to do with your life and the relative unimportance of eating a high-fat goopy dessert in the scheme of things. In larger parties, movement and standing rather than sitting can help in related ways. It expends more energy to stand rather than sit (approximately 20% more). It also keeps you focused on the people at the event and less on food.

- *Planning.* Planning is a key element of the heart and soul of the *Wellspring Plan*. A healthy obsession involves thinking in detailed ways about centrally important aspects of your life. Planning directs that thinking to something very constructive. It essentially sets a variety of goals about how you will handle something and what you will think about when you are in a high-risk situation. Planning also involves invoking images of yourself remaining focused, attentive, and effective as a weight controller. Finally, planning entails problem solving, such as making calls to hosts of parties or deciding whether or not to attend certain functions based on the people rather than the nature of the food or drink available.

- *Self-Monitoring.* This chapter focused on many critical ways in which self-monitoring deserves its place at the very center of the *Wellspring Plan.* When you self-monitor consistently, you evaluate and focus consistently. This process not only helps you cope with difficult situations, but allows you to reinforce the importance of your goals, both short-term and long-term. Consider the likely effect on you if you self-monitor each and every holiday meal. Would this make you more or less likely to eat with abandon in such high-risk situations? Committing to self-monitoring consistently should also reduce the amount of your quantitative deviations and decrease the frequency of any qualitative deviations from the *Wellspring Plan.*

These five strategies can enable you to manage any high-risk situation effectively. Research on lapsing and relapsing repeatedly shows that those who don't lapse try to do at least *something* when confronted with high-risk situations. Those who lapse just let the situation dominate their actions and thinking. Certainly as a committed participant in the *Wellspring Plan* you can occasionally go with the flow. That means that you can enjoy parties and being with friends and not planning every second of where your feet move from one point to the next. It does not mean that you relinquish your commitment to yourself and your program. You can have fun and be as comfortable in almost any situation without eating high-fat, greasy food. You can also record what you're eating in your head without making that a source of misery or discomfort. In fact, it might help to write down what you're eating at such events. That allows you to focus more on other things.

As you develop these incredibly important skills within your *Wellspring Plan*, you'll become increasingly comfortable with them. Over time, the use of these strategies will seem as natural to you as brushing your teeth at the end of the day or taking a shower in the morning. They just become part of your routine that allows you to negotiate your world healthfully and comfortably. They don't dominate or detract from your life if you use them consistently and effectively. Remaining overweight or continuing to gain and lose weight in rapidly repeating cycles, by quite dramatic contrast, decreases your chances of enjoying a comfortable life.

Step 7: Understand and Manage Stress— With and Without Food

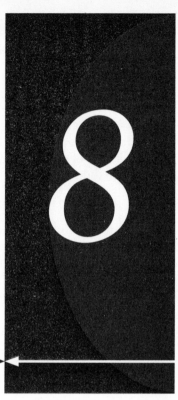

"[People] are disturbed not by things, but by the view which they take of them."

—EPICTETUS, First Century, *The Enchiridion*

THE PROBLEMS CAUSED BY deviating from the program by eating qualitatively poor foods go beyond immediate weight gain. If eating high-fat foods becomes an option when you're upset, those foods become even more desirable. You want those foods to become less desirable than they used to be for you—not sources of comfort. You want to view pizza with full-fat mozzarella cheese as too greasy. You want chocolate to seem too rich. At the very least, you want to train yourself to view all high-fat foods as "problematic." Let's consider the nature of stress and how you can manage stress without problematic foods.

Stress and Stressors: Definitions

This chapter will review sources of stress and consider methods of managing such challenging emotions using safe foods and methods other than eating. Please review Alice's and Maxine's stories (below). These stories illustrate one common source of stress, but two very different methods of coping. One approach maintains a healthful attitude (and weight); the other one does not.

ALICE'S ANXIETY

Alice had money trouble. She was a high school teacher and made a good living. But she had expensive tastes. She liked luxury cars, exotic vacations, and fine dining. Alice was divorced and had recently helped pay for her two children's college educations. The financial strain created by her penchant for expensive luxuries combined with college costs was affecting her every day. She found herself barely able to pay for necessities, falling behind on car payments and feeling beaten down by all of it.

Alice found that curling up on the couch and eating pizza, chips, and ice cream helped her escape her financial woes. When she munched, she worried less. She periodically tried dieting, but didn't maintain the attempts very long. She joined the YMCA a few blocks from her home, but rarely went there. Her weight steadily increased and her health and energy level declined.

Notice how Alice grappled with her money troubles through escape. She escaped to her couch, her movies, and her food. She had some moments when she sought change through action. But those actions were infrequent and quickly abandoned.

MAXINE'S CHALLENGE

Maxine had money trouble. She had just graduated from Northwestern University with a double-major in communication arts and drama. During college, she received financial help from her father, a scholarship, and government loans. Unfortunately, she received numerous credit cards in the mail and started using two of them.

Maxine had spent half of her senior year at Oxford University (England) and found more uses for money than she had known existed. Maxine and friends rented cars and toured Europe, played golf in Scotland, and had great mini-adventures. The credit card accounts swelled insidiously. Maxine's role in a local play didn't pay much (great experience, but not so great money).

Maxine graduated and decided to live in one of the world's priciest places: New York City. She thought she'd get a job, even waiting tables, and join the ranks of struggling actors—until she got her big break, of course. Meanwhile, her college loans and credit card debts began tightening their grip. She found herself worrying about paying basic bills every day.

Maxine had lost twenty unwanted pounds and gotten into the best shape of her life in England. She walked everywhere and ate a very low-fat diet (despite England's relatively high-fat cuisine). As her financial worries increased post-graduation, she noticed that she began eating more fast food, moving less, and regaining quite a few of those twenty pounds.

Maxine decided to do something constructive about her financial and physical struggles. She became a dog walker. She and another struggling artist created a Web site, put up signs, and started a little company called "Walk This Way." At first, the dog walking just supplemented her income as a server in a local diner. After a while, the word got out among canine aficionados that the "WTW Gals" were great. They hired other actors and artists, maintained their marketing campaign, and Maxine walked her way into a healthier body, as well as a financially more comfortable existence.

Both Alice and Maxine faced a similar source of unhappiness: lack of money. Both of them experienced stress, that is, complex negative emotional responses to a demand—a stressor—from the environment. How each woman dealt with such stress, however, is the key to their stories.

Types of Stressors

Stressors generally seem unpredictable and/or uncontrollable. Alice and Maxine faced money problems that had those qualities. Bills would appear that jarred them. They had felt they had their affairs in decent order when suddenly new bills would appear that their bank accounts couldn't handle. They'd use checks from one credit card to pay another; then they realized that their interest payments kept growing and growing.

Both major life events and daily hassles create stress. These stressors have unpredictable and uncontrollable elements. Did you ever move or change jobs and find that everything went according to your expectations? When you lost something, didn't it feel that your life was getting "out of control"?

Some examples of major life events include:

- Changing jobs
- Moving
- Conflict in a major relationship
- Serious illness or injury
- Death of a loved one

Some daily hassles include:

- Misplacing keys
- Being late
- Performing poorly at a task or a sport
- Failing to understand something
- Worrying about someone else's problems
- Weather problems
- Traffic problems
- Being criticized
- Forgetting something

You may have felt some discomfort just reading this list and remembering your reactions to events like these. Would it affect your food choices if you were late or if you were interrupted from completing something or if you were grappling with a major life event? Would your activity and exercise routines stay intact?

Certainly stressors challenge weight-control behaviors. If you can find more effective approaches to managing stressors, you'll become a more masterful weight controller.

Stress Management Techniques

Psychologists have studied stress management for decades and learned about those who barely survive versus those who prosper when faced with stressors. The Maxines in the world, like the athletes who perform well under pressure, are described as "resilient" or "hardy."

Resilience

Resilient (or hardy) people not only avoid harm from stressors, they often flourish under this type of pressure. Psychologist Suzanne Kobasa's research indicates that Three Cs describe how they do this: commitment, control, and challenge.

Commitment. Maxine faced her financial difficulty head-on. Because she was committed to living her life the best way she knew how, she sought solutions and continued to think about and act upon these thoughts until she came upon the dog-walking idea. She did not passively allow the uncomfortable quality of financial strain to overwhelm her.

Control. Maxine took control of the financial problem by creating new and better ways of earning money. In contrast, Alice merely escaped the problem through her couch, movies, and food. Maxine tried to influence what happened in her life by taking action. Alice did not attempt to influence or control her financial future aggressively. Maxine firmly believes she can control at least some important aspects of her world and take actions to solve problems as they emerge.

Challenge. Maxine clearly recognizes that change is a normal part of life. She views changes as opportunities that challenge her to grow. Alice behaved as if she feared change because she was afraid that she might not be able to handle it or overcome the difficulties of her financial condition. Alice attempted to just manage to survive the stressor she experienced rather than become more competent or skilled in a way that could help her overcome it. Maxine, on the other hand, sought a new solution and a new way to become more competent. Merely "adjusting" would bore her.

Various researchers have found that people like Maxine who are committed to their lives and work, who believe they can control their fates, and who see stressors as positive challenges manage stress quite effectively. Resilient lawyers and executives remain much healthier than their less hardy colleagues even when faced with many stressors.

Resilient weight controllers don't let setbacks or disappointments derail them. For example, if you gained a couple of pounds and had a poor day or week eating you could either give up and stop looking at the weight on a scale or you could take a more resilient approach. Resilient weight controllers will make sure to self-monitor, do more planning, and take additional steps to increase activity when problems arise. They don't stop looking at scales or looking at mirrors. They keep moving forward, committing to making a positive change in their lives and to looking at the many challenges of successful weight control as just that: challenges.

In general, to become more resilient, consider responding to stressors by asking yourself a few questions that direct you to take charge. For example:

- What can I do to eliminate this stressor?
- How can I look at this problem as an opportunity for change and growth?
- In what ways does this stressor teach me something about my life?
- How can I use this situation to improve my functioning or competence?

Becoming more resilient also involves a little help from your friends. Maxine was not alone when she began her dog-walking business. Maxine's family also cared about her and helped her make the change more smoothly. As discussed in the next section, family and friends can help a great deal—especially in the face of stressors.

Support from Your Friends & Family

People who have good relationships with others suffer fewer medical and emotional problems than more isolated people. People who get good support from others even live longer than those without good connections to other people. A study of seven thousand adults in Alameda County, California, for example, showed that people who lacked relationships with others died at a younger age than those who were married, had frequent contacts with friends and neighbors, and belonged to social clubs or religious groups.

As the study showed, support from others can reduce the effects of various stressors:

- Women who had another person with them during labor and childbirth experienced fewer complications than did women who did not have a husband, relative, or friend present. The supported group gave birth sooner, were awake more after delivery, and played with their babies more than the unsupported group.
- Social support helped men who lost their jobs. Men with good support reported fewer illnesses and less depression than men who did not have adequate support from others following the loss of their jobs.
- Support by parents and hospital staff helped children adjust more effectively to surgery.
- Recovery from heart attacks was improved when people had spouses, friends, and relatives around them.

How do your family and friends support you? How do they help? What do they give you or do for you? The way most people answer these questions indicates that they need more than just the presence of other people; they need people around who actively show that they care.

People show their support in three ways. Family and friends provide us with emotional comfort, helpful information, and material goods such as money or food. All three of these qualities of support can help you manage stress effectively.

Emotional Support. People provide emotional support when they:

- listen and talk things over when you want to feel that someone understands you
- allow you to talk freely about your problems and private thoughts
- show confidence in you and encourage you

Informational Support. People provide you with informational support when they:

- give you advice you can count on
- give you names of people who can do very competent work (good doctors and lawyers, for example)
- give you good ideas about personal and family problems

Material Support. People provide you with material support when they:

- look after your belongings (like plants or pets) if you have to leave town for a few days
- help you get to a doctor if you can't get yourself to one
- loan you money when you really need it

So, part of stress management includes knowing when and whom to ask for help. Can you identify who you can and do use for support among your family members, neighbors, and coworkers? Does your support network include especially good listeners and very reliable people? When life's little stressors increase, leaning on others helps. Friends and family can provide information, material goods, or emotional support, but their job of helping often becomes easier if we ask for the specific kind of help we want.

Sometimes when you ask for help, you don't get it. Social support doesn't always happen just because you have a spouse who "should" provide such support. Consider the case of Bob's problems with Pauline, presented below.

PROBLEMS WITH PAULINE—AND THEN FOOD

Bob and Pauline had been married for four tumultuous years. Pauline was a successful journalist for a major newspaper and Bob was an accountant at a large firm in the same city. They both had busy professional lives filled with demands and challenges. They often devoted more time to their professions than their relationship. They seemed to fight about almost everything, and food was no exception.

Bob decided to work conscientiously to improve his eating and exercising habits. He was approximately forty pounds overweight when he began this quest. Pauline was also somewhat overweight, but she did not want to make it a priority in her life. When Bob began eating lower-fat foods and making more and more time for exercising, Pauline objected. They began fighting about what to eat and, more specifically, about what Bob should eat. After several weeks of these skirmishes, Bob laid down the law to Pauline: "I am going to decide what I eat and you have to live with it. If I want your ideas about it, I'll ask. This is important to me and I want you to let me make these changes." Pauline conceded Bob's right to manage his own body. The skirmishes decreased and a peaceful, although somewhat uneasy, state emerged.

Over the course of the next year, Bob lost almost all of the forty pounds and became a committed exerciser. He used his health club membership very effectively. He found that exercising provided a good outlet for his stressful life. Bob often talked to Pauline about this and encouraged her to consider using this facility to help herself, as well. Pauline resisted and never accompanied Bob to the club.

One day Bob discovered that Pauline was having an affair with a man at her office. Bob's relationship with Pauline had never been great, but it had become a convenient alternative to loneliness. All of that changed very quickly. Bob saw Pauline's violation of their commitment to each other as a major and crushing disappointment. He and Pauline argued and fought in ugly ways. During this time, paying attention to food and exercising became "unimportant" to Bob. "Nothing else mattered. I just didn't care," he would say. He ate what was available and he "just didn't feel like" exercising anymore. It didn't take long for the weight to come back on and for the old habits to re-emerge in full force.

Perhaps your conflicts in key relationships were less dramatic than Pauline and Bob's; yet even minor disagreements between couples can produce critical lapses. In addition, many spouses try to meddle too much in the life of the weight controller. They may see the weight controller eating high-fat foods. They may notice the weight controller decrease his or her exercising for a few days. When family members use these observations to pressure the weight controller to get back on track, this usually backfires. "I'll show you!" can become a terrific motivator for eating cookies and ice cream.

Because many families have problems with meddling, interfering, or trying to "help too much," I developed the guidelines below for spouses and family members. You may find it useful to photocopy this list to give to your spouse or family members. This information gently shows significant others how to help without interfering:

TABLE 8.1
HOW TO SUPPORT A WEIGHT CONTROLLER'S EFFORTS
Losing weight and keeping it off is a very difficult process. You can make it easier for your spouse, friend, or partner. Here are several suggestions that will help you support and encourage the weight controllers in your life:
General Attitude
Be positive. Convey to the weight controller that even though it is very difficult to control weight, you believe he or she can do it. This attitude will boost the person's self-confidence while acknowledging the difficulties. Avoid negative comments, criticism, and coercion. These are unhelpful and demoralizing and will create negative feelings between you and the weight controller. This, in turn, could cause him or her to eat more—not less—and could thwart the likelihood of success in the long run.

TABLE 8.1 (CONTINUED)
HOW TO SUPPORT A WEIGHT CONTROLLER'S EFFORTS

General Attitude (continued)

Be reinforcing. Acknowledge the weight controller's accomplishments. Compliments, attention, encouragement, and tangible reinforcement (like little gifts) can help him or her stay motivated and adhere to the plan. Remember, be sincere; superficiality will be interpreted as condescending and aversive.

Be realistic. Weight control requires tremendous effort and skill to overcome strong biological forces. People who are trying to lose weight must adopt eating and exercise patterns that are much more stringent than normal. Don't expect the weight controller to be perfect, or even close to perfect. Occasional slips of overeating, inactivity, weight gain, and failure to adhere to plans will occur. Help the weight controller learn from these experiences rather than dwell on them as "failures."

Communicate. Occasionally inquire about the weight controller's progress. Ask him or her how you can help, thereby complementing the weight controller's individual efforts. Be open to discussing the challenges of weight control and to assist in solving problems.

Managing Food

Increase the amount of nutritious, low-fat foods available to the weight controller.

Do not encourage the weight controller to eat foods that he or she is trying to avoid (for example, refrain from saying, "Let's go out for ice cream," or "Oh, come on, a little bit isn't going to hurt you").

Help the weight controller prepare foods and recipes in a low-fat way. Encourage experimentation and adventure.

Adopt appropriate eating habits, for example: not eating when full, eating appropriate portions, eating slowly, eating regularly or on a schedule, limiting snacking, and limiting the number of eating situations. You may not have a weight problem, but better eating habits may improve your health and will support the weight controller's efforts.

Plan activities with the weight controller that do not revolve around food (for example, sporting events, concerts, games).

When you go to a restaurant with the weight controller, select places that make low-fat/low-sugar eating as pleasant as possible.

Promoting Exercise

Plan activities with the weight controller that involve exercise (for example, walking, hiking, sports).

Become an exercise partner. You will reap the same physical benefits as your partner.

Support and encourage the weight controller's individual efforts to exercise.

You can't expect your significant others to provide the kind of support suggested in the above list without lapsing, occasionally, back into their former patterns. When this occurs, as it inevitably does, you will do yourself the most good by handling it in a gentle and understanding manner. For example, if your spouse becomes a bit negative or criticizes a food choice that you made, *try to avoid an angry outburst.* Instead, try saying something like, "I don't think it helps me when you are negative like that. Remember, no one does weight control perfectly."

Your sources of support also require some maintenance from you. It is very important to give as well as receive support. To do this, you may wish to look for signs from others that they feel stressed. Try to notice when your friends and key family members reach out in your direction. They may start calling you more often or asking you to spend time with them. You may even feel annoyed about having to manage their requests for your time and attention while you are busy with your own problems. When feeling such annoyance, think about responding positively to their efforts as depositing money in a savings account. Providing support for your significant others when they need it, even when such efforts add stress to your life, can pay off with a huge dividend when you find yourself needing help.

Stress Inoculation

Psychologist Don Meichenbaum developed a useful approach to handling major stressors. This technique, called stress inoculation, builds "psychological antibodies." Physical antibodies are microscopic particles in our bloodstreams that attack foreign substances like bacteria. Stress inoculation has helped people prevent and attack problematic emotions like anger and anxiety, improving test-taking, social skills, anxiety from public speaking, anxiety associated with performing music, and fear of flying. It can help you improve your weight control. The procedure includes an educational phase and a coping self-talk phase.

Education about the Stressor. In this phase of stress inoculation, important information about the stressor is provided. For example, children going to their first dental appointment may not know what happens there. A friend may have told them that it hurts or that a big person in a white coat will yank out their teeth with a pair of pliers. Just learning what happens in a real dental visit often helps young patients adapt to that difficult situation. In a similar way, many people lack information about a variety of stressors. Students often do not know the best strategies for taking tests; medical patients often have serious misconceptions about their illnesses or about hospitals and treatments; and, more generally, people often do not ask enough questions to learn about new jobs, new cities, new cars, and other potentially stressful events.

When facing a stressor, you will benefit if you ask questions of people who do understand it, read about it, and take other actions to educate yourself about its nature and effects.

Coping Self-Statements. All people talk to themselves sometimes. You may have noticed that you talk yourself into doing difficult things. Imagine taking your first dive off a diving board or making your first public speech. You may recall making self-statements like "C'mon, you can do it," "You know what to do," and "Go for it." These statements provide instructions and encouragement that help when facing challenges of all kinds.

Psychologists advise people facing such challenges to use four types of self-statements: preparing for the stressor, confronting and handling the stressor, coping with feelings at critical moments, and rewarding oneself for successful coping. The following lists provide examples of these four types of self-statements that you can use to manage almost any stressor. As you can see by the lists, people who use these self-statements actively cope with stressors. This approach encourages you to become a "hardy" or resilient coper. Both approaches to stress management encourage you to see stressors as opportunities to exert control and to enjoy and benefit from a challenge.

Think of a stressor you recently faced. It could be taking an exam, going to a doctor or dentist, asking for a favor, or talking in front of a group of people. Try to imagine how you would talk yourself into and through these challenges. Then review the list of self-statements below and see if you could have used some of them to help you manage that stressor.

SELF-STATEMENTS WHEN PREPARING FOR A STRESSOR
- What do I have to do?
- I can create a plan to deal with this.
- Thinking about what I have to do is certainly better than getting nervous about it.
- Worrying won't help. Plan.
- My anxiety tells me that I have a challenge facing me.
- I can learn from this.
- Remain logical and calm.

SELF-STATEMENTS WHEN CONFRONTING AND HANDLING THE STRESSOR

- I can handle this.
- I can meet this challenge.
- Just take it one step at a time; follow the plan.
- Beat the fear: think of what I am doing.
- Relax. I'm in control. Just take a slow, deep breath.
- My tension just tells me to follow my plan; deal with this challenge.
- I can eat safe foods as part of my plan.

SELF-STATEMENTS WHEN COPING WITH FEELINGS AT CRITICAL MOMENTS

- When tension comes, just pause and breathe slowly.
- Focus on the present. Now, what do I have to do?
- I've handled this before and I can manage it now.
- I'll rate my fear from one to ten and then watch it change.
- I'll just keep the tension manageable; I won't worry about eliminating it altogether.
- I can do this. It will be over in a certain amount of time.
- Okay, keep focused on what I want to do.
- This is not the worst thing that can happen.
- Remember, I don't have to handle this perfectly, just reasonably well.
- Focus on sensations: coldness, warmth, smells, touch, taste, sights, and sounds.
- Think about other times and places. Good feelings come with good thoughts.
- I'm in control.
- If I'm going to overeat, I'll deviate quantitatively, not qualitatively.

SELF-STATEMENTS WHEN REWARDING YOURSELF FOR SUCCESSFUL COPING

- Nice going! I was able to do it.
- It wasn't as tough as I expected.
- Wait 'til I tell [a friend, spouse, or other family member] about it.
- I'm making progress.
- My plan worked.
- I'm learning all the time.
- It's my thinking that creates tension. When I control my self-

statements, I can control my tension.
- I'm doing better each time I use these self-statements.
- I'm really pleased with my progress.

Weight controllers face many stressors that can directly impact their efforts to either lose weight or maintain a low weight. For example, consider the impact of going to a party. Parties include lots of high-fat food, alcoholic drinks, and people in a generally relaxed and unrestrained state. Some parties also go on late into the evening, increasing your feelings of tiredness. Parties also include people who might encourage you to eat or drink in problematic ways. How could you use the stress inoculation approach to handle this stressor?

First, the educational aspect of stress inoculation would encourage you to find out all you can about the event. The following are several questions my clients ask to educate themselves about parties before going to them:

- How many people will be there?
- What kind of food will be served?
- More specifically, are there options for the main course and are there good (safe) options during the hors d'oeuvres or early phases of the party?
- Will there be people there with whom I would like to talk and spend time?
- Will I be bored?
- Will I be able to leave when I feel like it?

The answers to these questions determine whether the situation will create a major or minor challenge to your weight-control efforts. If low-fat options abound and if the people will provide good distractions, the situation becomes easier to manage. On the other hand, a boring party combined with abundant high-fat food may require you to cope at a high level.

Coping self-statements could help you get through challenging parties. For example, you could try some of the following ideas:

Preparing:
- I can create a plan that will get me through this.
- I don't have to worry about this; I can plan for it.

- I'm sure I can learn from this and get even better at managing these kinds of situations.
- Plan:
  - Get a diet drink or a sparkling water and hang on to it.
  - Find the most interesting people available and talk with them.
  - Convince my spouse to leave if I give him/her the signal.
  - Make the "signal" dramatic, like "We have to go now, dear!" if necessary.

Confronting and handling:
- I can handle this.
- There are a lot of people here, but that gives me greater choices.
- Stay focused and remember: Everything counts!

Coping at critical moments:
- If I see some tempting morsel in the hors d'oeuvres phase, I'll grip my drink even more tightly.
- Remember to find some low-fat alternatives; they've got to be here.
- Even if I eat some problematic foods, I can still count it and record it.
- Every food has finite calories and fat grams; nothing is going to kill me here.
- Let me find somebody I can talk to who can make me laugh.
- I can get something else to drink that is healthier.
- Even if the main course is chock full of problems, I don't have to eat a lot of it.

Reward myself for success:
- Nice going. I basically followed the plan.
- The plan was good even though I did eat a few things I didn't want to.
- I think I'm getting better at this.

Weight control requires a degree of obsessiveness (healthy obsessiveness, that is). You have to concentrate intently when facing stressors, particularly stressors that can directly impact your weight control efforts. If you can accept the requirement of this extra concentration, you can use it as a personal challenge. Stressors can also help you learn about yourself and help you become more of a master of your own fate.

Relaxation Techniques

The box below shows some examples of "cued relaxation." This technique encourages you to include relaxation as part of your everyday life. By using the cues that you find in your normal environment to remind yourself to take a relaxation break, you can prevent little hassles from becoming big stressors.

CUED RELAXATION

Instructions

Find some cues from your everyday life you can use to remind you to take brief relaxation breaks. Such cues could include the ringing of your telephone, drinking water from a fountain, reaching for your wallet, or combing your hair. When the cue occurs, take a few seconds to use a relaxation technique.

Examples:

Cue = Phone Call

1. Phone rings.
2. Answer the phone.
3. Use a breathing technique (e.g., slow rhythmic breathing).
4. During the call focus on breathing in a relaxed manner.
5. After the phone call, take another few seconds to execute the relaxation technique once again.

Cue = Drinking Water or Coffee

1. Begin drinking.
2. Focus on the fluid and the sounds and sights of it.
   - What color is it?
   - What does it sound like specifically as you drink?
   - Concentrate on the texture of the fluid as it enters your mouth and goes down your throat.
3. Create a vivid image that involves water. For example:
   - You are on a beach in the summertime and you are watching a lake gently flow to the shore and retreat from the shore.
   - You are hiking on a mountain and you come upon a beautiful waterfall. You are watching the water flow and beat down on the rocks below. You are listening to the sounds and smelling the air.
   - Take a few minutes to stay in the image, keeping it vivid, using all of your senses to enliven the imagery.

Cue = Reaching for Your Wallet

1. After your hand makes contact with the wallet, remind yourself to relax.
2. Tense and then relax some of the muscles in your hand and arm. Tense and relax those muscles at least twice.
3. Pay attention to the change in sensation from the tense to the relaxed state for each muscle group that you use. Focus on the relaxed state for a few seconds and try to bring that sense of relaxation from the top of your head through your eyes and down to the rest of your body.

Detailed Plans for Coping with Three Common Stressors

Three stressors in particular consistently contribute to the stress experienced by weight controllers: travel, holidays, and restaurants. Let's consider some specialized plans and coping responses that you may find more useful than the more basic discussion of these situations presented in the last chapter.

Travel

"When I go on my business trips to the East, I know exactly which places I like for meals and snacks. Unfortunately, most of the stuff is junk food. I know where the Pizza Huts are. I know where the Häagen-Dazs shops are. I even know where to get seemingly healthy, but high-fat, trail mixes. I seem drawn to these places when I travel. Somehow I convince myself that I need a break today. It's been a long frustrating day. It's okay to eat X, Y, Z."

Does this sound familiar? Traveling produces many frustrations and little control. We don't know which plane is going to be late, where our luggage will wind up and what food will be available at what times of the day. In addition, our usual patterns of eating are thrown to the wind by dehydration, jet lag, and changes in time zones. Many people also sleep less soundly when they travel. This produces yet another type of altered state: fatigue. Our normal schedules are thrown off *and* we have to face easily available high-fat, high-sugar foods—quite a challenging combination!

Some of the problems when flying begin in the airplane itself. First, airplanes are kept extremely dry. It is critical to drink at least one glass of non-caffeinated fluid for every hour you spend in flight. Consider bringing a bottle of water with you on the plane. This can improve your sense of control as it prevents dehydration. If you rely on flight attendants to get the fluid you need, you may become both dehydrated and frustrated if they are slow or unavailable.

Another major source of the problems that occur when flying concerns the food. Remember, peanuts get 69 to 93% calories from fat. They also contain 166 calories in a one-ounce packet. That's a lot of fat and a lot of calories in one or two quick bites. Alcoholic drinks also cause the body to lose water, exacerbating the already difficult fluid problem. They also reduce restraint. This can pave the way for high-calorie eating and snacking.

The in-flight meals and snack boxes, now available for purchase on many flights, are perhaps the most notorious problem about flying. Many of those small and sometimes very unappealing in-flight meals or snacks really seem like snacks. But they often contain six hundred or more calories, many of which come from fat. The boredom of flying makes these little unappealing snacks seem much more appealing. Many people also proceed to have a full meal soon after arriving at their destinations.

The simplest way to manage airline food is to avoid it entirely. In recent years, many more people bring their own foods on planes. Just pack a meal that will work for your eating plan. It helps to include some snack items (like pretzels, low-fat popcorn, fruit, vegetables) to help ameliorate the boredom of the trip.

Here are a few other travel tips for frequent flyers:

- Try to minimize the fat in the standard airline meal or snack. For example, when the flight attendant brings you the food, hand back the margarine, high-fat salad dressing, and dessert. Simply give these items to the attendant and make as minimal a comment as you would like. You are not required to justify making healthy food choices if you do not wish to.
- Remove the skin from chicken and scrape away any gravies or sauces.
- Bring low-fat snack foods with you. Raisins, crackers, cereal, and pretzels may provide good alternatives to some of the snacks available. (The tricky part is to wait until you are in the air before munching.)
- Try to plan your meals carefully on the days you travel. For example, if you schedule a lunch or a dinner meeting when you arrive, consider turning down the in-flight snack. This would be a good time to use your own low-calorie snack or meal.

Traveling by air presents many challenges, but so does traveling by car, bus, or train. All modes of travel create irregularities in schedules and moods. Many of my clients and I have found it particularly helpful to exercise in the morning before traveling. This provides some stress relief and makes it more tolerable to sit for hours. Another key remedy for the travails of travel is planning. That is, by carefully (even obsessively) planning your traveling, you can avoid some of the common pitfalls. Weight controllers who plan their meals carefully and ensure that low-fat, low-calorie snacks are available, for example, take some of the risk out of traveling. Weight controllers who have reached the Acceptance stage often lose weight while traveling. They use traveling as an opportunity to seek out activity and to avoid the temptations of readily accessible refrigerators and cupboards.

Yet another challenge imposed by traveling concerns people. Consider Al:

AL'S SOUTHERN CHALLENGE

"I am Jewish and was born and raised in Chicago, the city that works: the city with Big Shoulders. Emphasis on *big*. My wife grew up in Memphis, Tennessee, and she's Christian. Her parents, grandparents, and all of her relatives are from the really far South—emphasis on *South*. You could say we are from different worlds—because we are.

I've made huge changes in the way I eat and in the way I exercise. I've really been working at this for three and a half years now and I've lost fifty pounds. I still want to lose another fifty and I'm getting there. It's a struggle every day, but I'm getting there. My wife weighs eighty pounds less than I do and eats more food and calories every day than I do. Most people find that hard to believe, but it's true. She eats desserts several times per week. I almost never do. She eats fried foods occasionally. I don't. I exercise all the time, she almost never does. It's just the biological breaks, I guess.

Well, this plays out in a pretty funny way when we go to visit her relatives in Tennessee. I don't think many of the people who live in the southern part of the United States have quite gotten into the low-fat eating business. At least my wife's relatives sure haven't. They eat ham practically for every meal! Butter, biscuits, gravy, country ham, regular ham, mayonnaise, cakes, fried everything.

I've known these fine people for more than ten years now. I've just really confused them in the last three. They don't know how to feed me anymore, and it presents certain challenges for all of us. For example, after we get to my wife's aunt's house, which is where we sometimes stay for weekends when we visit with her family, I immediately go to the grocery store. I stock up on skim milk, fresh vegetables, no-salt pretzels, and a few other mainstays. They've learned that I just won't eat certain things. They've made a real effort to have raw vegetables available for me and cook some foods that for them are unusual (like chicken instead of ham). They even go so far as to buy apples occasionally or some other snack food that I can eat. Unfortunately, the apples they buy don't quite meet my Chicago standards most of the time—they're usually rather anemic and bumpy. But it's a nice thought! They even avoid buttering and putting bacon fat on vegetables—quite a change for these people.

I make sure I exercise every day when I visit there. Sometimes this means getting up before my small children wake up, even if it's before the sun peeks out over the hills. This usually makes me tired, but it allows me to stay with the program in a difficult situation. These folks definitely try to get me to eat, and they sometimes make fun of me for my 'strange ways.' I try not to make a big deal out of it. We seem to have adjusted to each other reasonably well."

Al effectively asserted himself with his relatives. Family members can be food-pushers. Food is a complex commodity. People use it to express themselves. Food can also be used to control situations and other people. Getting people to overeat helps some people feel less guilty about their own problematic habits. It is helpful to realize that traveling involves negotiating and asserting yourself with other people. The central question for you when you travel is: *do you have the right to eat in a healthy, effective way wherever you are*? (The answer is YES!).

Holidays

Thanksgiving is a classic holiday that many Americans consider a well-justified eating orgy. Actually, in the following Thanksgiving dinner menu, you can see that many of the elements of the classic Thanksgiving meal are healthy foods:

Foods/Serving Size	Calories
Turkey (no skin, one-half white, one-half dark meat) - 3 ounces	148
Mashed potatoes - 1 cup	222
Gravy - ½ cup	61
Stuffing - ½ cup	250

Candied sweetpotato - 1	144
Cranberry sauce - 2 tablespoons	52
Fresh fruit salad - ½ cup	62
Celery - 1 stalk	5
Carrots - ½ cup	15
Bread - 1 roll	71
Butter - 1 pat	35
White wine - ½ cup	80
Pumpkin pie - 1 slice	300
Whipped cream - ¼ cup	200
Coffee	0
Total	**1,645**

The white meat turkey without the skin, potatoes, fresh fruit salad, celery and carrots, and even white wine pose no major problems. It's the stuffing, gravy, butter, pumpkin pie crust, and whipped cream that pile on the calories and the excess fat. The meal listed above derives 21% of its calories from fat. By selecting the low-fat components of the classic Thanksgiving dinner, you could have a perfectly satisfactory meal.

My colleagues and I have found that weight controllers who are focused and plan their Thanksgiving holiday usually cope with it quite well. First, the food is predictable. Second, the company or social aspects of the situation are predictable and possibly controllable. If you are serving the feast, you can invite people with whom you want to talk. If you are going somewhere else, you can spend your time with the people who are interesting and enjoyable. Finally, remember that Thanksgiving is finite. It has a clear beginning and end. It doesn't go on and on for days with parties galore, as does Christmas.

The Christmas season poses greater risks for weight controllers. Unlike Thanksgiving, Christmas festivities last well beyond one particular day. There are pre-Christmas parties and mini-celebrations. There are sugary "treats" at the office. There are baking Christmas cookies and other rituals associated with high-fat, high-sugar foods. And, of course, this endless stream of parties can last for several weeks, including New Year's Eve. Alcohol also flows freely during this time of the year. Many restraints are lost and replaced instead by the "holiday spirit." All of this goes on during a time of the year when the coldness of the climate in many parts of the United States makes exercising especially challenging.

Easter and other holidays pose somewhat similar problems. These holidays also involve sugary and high-fat foods. They last quite a while, and restraint often yields to the holiday spirit.

Not surprisingly, many people gain weight during the holiday season (from Thanksgiving to New Year's). Weight controllers may gain even more weight than the average person because of their biological predispositions toward weight gain. Weight controllers can also lose the positive momentum that they may have developed prior to the holiday season. Getting back into low-fat, low-sugar eating and intensive frequent exercising once you take a vacation from it is a major psychological challenge. I've seen many people become derailed during the holiday season and take many months, sometimes years, to get back on track.

Several tricks of the trade are used by successful weight controllers during the holidays. Consider the following suggestions:

• **Plan Ahead**. When you plan ahead, you can predict and control your world. For example, think about your next party. Who's going to be there and what kind of food will be served? You can call your host and get a preview of the menu. You can make a tentative list of what you will eat, with whom you will talk, and how you will stay focused. It is particularly important to attempt to monitor your food record during the holiday season.

• **Avoid Starvation before a Celebration**. Starving before a big holiday meal can produce binge-eating. Starving produces deprivation and a very strong biological response to the sight of food. This biological response includes the secretion of insulin and saliva. In other words, if you eat nothing or very little before a big holiday meal or party, you will get incredibly hungry. This reaction is more likely to lead to problematic eating than controlled eating. An alternative approach would include selecting low-fat, low-sugar foods for breakfast and lunch. Having a small snack just before leaving for the party may help as well.

• **Scope Out the Food Scene**. After arriving, you can quickly survey the available options. Perhaps you will notice that there are fresh vegetables and other munchies that will work for you. You also can discover the main course will keep you on a low-fat, low-sugar plan. This scoping may prevent you from eating high-fat snacks such as chips, dips, nuts, and party mixes.

• **Use a Food Plan.** Once you are aware of the available and planned party foods, you can develop a specific food plan for what you will eat and a way of focusing on that plan. You can hold a glass of diet soft drink or water and keep your attention on the conversation instead of the food. You can also use this cue or some other cue (perhaps munching a raw vegetable) to remind yourself of your immediate goals and your long-range goals.

• **Refocus Your Holiday Season.** This suggestion goes well beyond an individual event or party. Holidays are traditionally focused around food and celebrations. You can break that tradition. You can focus on other people, special projects, and finding new, creative ways to relax. Some people develop their skills in winter sports and others focus on enjoying crackling fireplaces and reading some good books.

Restaurants

> At the Hearthside [Diner], we utilize whatever bit of autonomy we have to ply our customers with the illicit calories that signal our love. It is our job as servers to assemble the salads and desserts, pour the dressings, and squirt the whipped cream. We also control the number of butter pats our customers get and the amount of sour cream on their baked potatoes. So if you wonder why Americans are so obese, consider the fact that waitresses both express their humanity and earn their tips through the covert distribution of fats.
>
> —BARBARA EHRENREICH, *Nickel and Dimed in America*, p. 20.

Americans ate 25% of their meals outside of their homes in 1975. In 2009, it is estimated that Americans will probably eat 50% of their meals outside of their homes. Restaurant meals account for almost 50% of every dollar Americans spend on food. Americans eat 25% of their restaurant meals at fast-food eateries such as McDonald's, Burger King, Wendy's, or Pizza Hut.

You probably noticed that you, too, eat out more often now than ever before in your life. Restaurants offer the advantages of keeping you away from preparing food and the urge to nibble as you cook. On the other hand, restaurants often cook in mysterious ways, using more fat and more sugar than you would to prepare food. Some eateries can also lull you into making problematic food choices because of their style or atmosphere.

It requires clarity of thinking and assertiveness to eat healthfully in restaurants.

It is your *right* to request that the food you order at a restaurant is prepared according to your wishes, your right to get what you pay for. Most restaurateurs want to accommodate their patrons. In a recent survey conducted by MasterCard, more than 90% of the restaurateurs who were surveyed said they preferred hearing complaints about orders directly. They want you to be satisfied and to bring your business back to them. Still, some servers resist providing you with the information you want about food preparation. Remind yourself of your right to that information, then try making a polite request, even repeated requests, if necessary. This strategy should work well most of the time. For example:

PATRON: "I'll take the chicken dish with broccoli and new potatoes. How is that prepared?"
SERVER: "How is what prepared?"
PATRON: "The chicken."
SERVER: "I think it's broiled."
PATRON: "In other words, it might be sautéed instead of broiled?"
SERVER: "Yeah."
PATRON: "Could you check on that for me, please?"
SERVER: "Okay."
(Server leaves for two minutes to check on preparation of the chicken and then returns.)
SERVER: "It's broiled."
PATRON: "Great. Then I'll go with the chicken. I'd like the vegetables grilled, with no butter added on them."
SERVER: "I don't think they put any butter on the vegetables or the potatoes."
PATRON: "Please be sure that no butter or any sauces are added to the broccoli or the potatoes, okay?"
SERVER: "Okay."

Does this patron seem overly pushy to you? If you answered "yes," you still have a problem. Remember, you have the right to get what you pay for. That includes knowing what you're getting. If your server does not comply with reasonable requests for this kind of information, you could ask to speak to the manager or the owner. You could also leave the restaurant. What does not work is to stay and eat foods that you want to avoid.

Sometimes my clients lament the limited choices in certain types of restaurants. One of my clients countered these laments eloquently: "I can always find *something* to eat." He meant that he could always find something to eat that fits well with his weight control program. Perhaps even he would be challenged by the notoriously limited menus in small-town bars, but for the most part his view coincides with that of virtually all successful weight controllers. Consider some of the options below for a variety of ethnic restaurants:

- **Cajun.** Seafood or vegetable gumbo or jambalaya (without sausage), grilled fish.
- **Chinese.** First, ask what can be prepared without oil. Stir-fries prepared with fat-free sauces, broths, or soy sauce; chicken, seafood, and vegetables; soups (hot and sour, chicken, vegetable); chicken and shrimp dishes steamed without sauces.
- **French.** Poached, grilled, or steamed fish; chicken and wine sauce; Nicoise salads without oil.
- **Greek.** Chicken and fish shish kebabs; salads, couscous, rice.
- **Indian.** Tandoori chicken, prawns, fish.
- **Italian.** Pasta with red clam sauce, meatless marinara; pizza with no cheese and steamed vegetable toppings; minestrone soup (made without butter).
- **Japanese.** Sushi, chicken and fish teriyaki, tofu and vegetables (avoid avocado, mayonnaise, eel, and mackerel).
- **Mexican.** Chicken and seafood enchiladas with no cheese; tamales with no cheese; chicken or shrimp fajitas (without sour cream, guacamole) and made with "as little oil as possible"; chicken taco salad (no cheese); salsa (request tortillas as a side dish to dip into salsa instead of chips).
- **Thai.** First, ask "What can you prepare without oil?" Then, stir-fried shrimp, chicken, and vegetable dishes can work for you. Also, soups, especially sweet and sour (Tom Yun) soup; chicken and cucumber salads.

A critical saying to remember when ordering food in restaurants is: *If you don't know what the food is or how it was prepared, assume the worst!* This saying directs you to find something on the menu that you can rely on. If you look diligently enough on virtually every menu, you, too, "can always find something to eat."

"There's nothing either good or bad but thinking makes it so."
—WILLIAM SHAKESPEARE, *Hamlet*

Step 8: Use Slump Busters to Overcome Slumps

MOST WEIGHT CONTROLLERS begin a new weight loss effort fueled considerably by past frustrations. This often creates a Honeymoon stage, even with low-carb diets and other misguided approaches. As you read about in an earlier chapter and have probably discovered for yourself, the Honeymoon stage usually leads to the much more challenging Frustration stage. Even if you blasted through your Frustration stage and settled more comfortably in an Acceptance stage in your *Wellspring Plan*, you still face the biggest challenge of them all: *time*.

Time can work for you or against you in weight control. Usually, it does both. Time helps you by cementing your new habits into a lifestyle that becomes increasingly clear and solid. Highly successful weight controllers report that the *Wellspring Plan* gets significantly easier at three years post-weight loss than at one year and easier still at six years versus three. Your biology cooperates, a little, with decreased stomach size and decreased preferences for high-fat foods. Master weight controllers also know where to shop to get their preferred low-fat foods (e.g., fat-free cheeses or fat-free frozen yogurt treats) and what to order at favorite restaurants. Patterns of high activity and exercise also become more ingrained, with greater levels of dissatisfaction when they are not followed.

Time works against you by eventually exposing you to all of the potential causes of slumps. As the days, weeks, and years tick by, stuff happens. Donna's story below illustrates this point. If forewarned is forearmed, then let's forewarn you by reviewing the nine most likely threats to your *Wellspring Plan* in the long run. Then, we'll examine seven approaches for strengthening your *Wellspring Plan* and getting the help you might need to bust those slumps, fast and forever. You can apply many of the first several slump busters quite easily to see if they get you back to the *Wellspring Plan*. If not, the final few ideas add more external structure to give you more support as you regenerate an effective *Wellspring Plan*. Remember that almost all weight controllers struggle to master their resistant biologies over time, at least occasionally. Those who develop true mastery of this most challenging of human quests learn how to anticipate slumps and take the necessary steps to overcome them. They refuse to give in to inertia or resistant biology.

DONNA'S DOUGHNUT

Donna was a twenty-six-year-old graduate student when she sought my help for her extra seventy-five-pound lifelong weight problem. As she was preparing her brain for a professional career (as a psychologist), she wanted to get her body ready for what she described as "the real world" (as opposed to life in a university).

She developed a wonderful *Wellspring Plan* with detailed self-monitoring and great consistency in eating, activity, and tenacity. She lost every pound that had plagued her, got a new wardrobe, and felt great about the transformation.

After losing the weight in seven months and maintaining her *Wellspring Plan* for another six, she came upon a doughnut one day during a contentious meeting with colleagues. By this time, Donna had finished her doctorate and moved to Philadelphia—and to a new life.

That first doughnut, the first in almost two years for Donna, somehow led her to the first high-fat muffin the very next day. Moreover, Donna's activity pattern had declined in her new life. She didn't find a convenient (and affordable) health club to replace the university gym she used almost every day when she was in graduate school. As Donna's eating patterns eroded, her steps decelerated as well. Donna's extra billions of fat cells couldn't have been happier—as they began refilling in Philly.

Nine Major Challenges

Drs. Roy Baumeister, Todd Heatherton, and Dianne Tice described the concept of "strength of self-regulation" in their important book *Losing Control: How and Why People Fail at Self-Regulation*. They noted that for those who have self-regulated effectively (by developing a *Wellspring Plan* and losing weight with this approach, for example) life events can overpower your self-regulation strength at times. They described studies that show that it takes energy to stay focused on self-regulation. For example, it takes time and energy for you to self-monitor, shop for fat-free foods, exercise, and use your pedometer. If your life becomes very hectic or changes in important ways, the energy used for the *Wellspring Plan* may become diverted to other things.

We'll consider in the final section of this chapter seven methods for improving the strength of your *Wellspring Plan*, your efficiency as a self-regulator, and other approaches to bolster the *Wellspring Plan* when the going gets rough. For now, let's review nine challenges that can threaten this new lifestyle you've developed. Understanding these challenges may help you anticipate and manage them more effectively.

Lapse Versus Relapse

The biology of excess weight makes it *impossible* for anyone to eat perfectly. Those hungry fat cells and associated hormones make an occasional French fry or doughnut virtually irresistible. So you need to view a *lapse* as a temporary problem, a temporary detour from the overall plan. In other words, lapsing does not have to lead to relapsing—that is, a full-blown change back into old, problematic styles of behavior.

Successful weight controllers persist in the face of the inevitable lapses. They realize that an occasional doughnut or ice cream cone is simply a mistake, not a catastrophe. They view these deviations as tolerable, not earth-shaking. Lapses become relapses when you discontinue self-monitoring of your eating and exercising. If you eat four pieces of pizza and consider it a disaster, you may give up monitoring for that day, that week, or that year. If you eat the pizza and consider it a problem to be solved, you can maintain your healthy obsession and continue making progress.

When solving the problem, you first have to deal with the reality of the event. That means calculating the cost to your progress of eating that pizza. For example, you figure that four pieces of pizza would have eighty fat grams, so you write that down and realize that eighty is not a million. Then you could analyze the situation you were in and try to consider ways of avoiding the problem the next time it presents itself. In this case, you could have taken the cheese and toppings off the pizza and eaten the bread with the remaining tomato sauce. So the lapse would have involved perhaps eight to ten fat grams, instead of eighty.

Two things to remember about lapses and relapses:

- Lapses are inevitable.
- Lapses don't become relapses if you maintain your consistent self-monitoring.

Injuries and Illnesses

Momentum is a magical thing. In weight control, you can build momentum for change. You can get into routines and rely on those routines to keep you going. Those routines are the lifeblood of your *Wellspring Plan*. Twisted ankles, bad backs, the flu, colds, and other problems can kill momentum by changing your routines.

Poorly managed injuries and illnesses can kill momentum for effective weight control. For example, one of my clients, David, developed chronic sinus infections after the birth of his second child. Children bring a lot of joy into life—but a lot of colds as well. David had allergy problems, but his children's "gift" of frequent colds increased his problems. Sinus infections are like mild colds that also produce fevers and sluggishness. Unfortunately, they don't go away in seven days. They tend to stick around for weeks or months if untreated by antibiotics. David found it difficult to maintain his jogging program and thereby control his weight because of these sinus infections.

He went to see an ear, nose, and throat specialist and an allergist. After a variety of tests, David's doctors decided the best course of action for him was to use very strong doses of antibiotics and also to "take it easier, listen to your body, and don't exercise so much."

Weight controllers also experience injuries. As you become more active in the *Wellspring Plan*, even by increasing your steps consistently, overuse injuries will occur occasionally. Your back could become strained or you could develop knee, hip, or foot problems. These momentum busters pose very real challenges. Athletes push their bodies hard. Successful weight controllers push their bodies hard as well.

Scale Phobia

"I didn't want to get on a scale this week because I think I gained weight." Does this sound familiar? It's a problematic attitude that can lead to lapses and slumps. Scales provide critical information to weight controllers that can assist in setting goals and changing patterns associated with weight gain.

Vacations

Most people find vacations relaxing, distracting, and enjoyable. Vacations are also dangerous to weight controllers. Vacations interfere with momentum. Vacations, like injuries and illnesses, cause changes in your usual routines. One of my clients, Renee, said, "I get into a 'vacation mentality.' The vacation mentality gets me to relax my restraint. I take it easy on myself. I don't force myself to exercise or count calories. I focus on my family and have fun." You can see that a "vacation mentality" can become a dangerous thing. Vacations can lead to decreases in exercise and re-emergence of higher-fat, higher-sugar eating. Once these patterns re-emerge, they become hard to kill off again.

Changes in Key Relationships

Major conflicts in key relationships can interfere with your life more dramatically than almost anything else. What happened to you the last time you had a major conflict at work? Most people report trouble sleeping and tremendous preoccupation when such conflicts occur. Conflicts at home produce even more dramatic symptoms. Major lapses can quickly become slumps during periods of conflict with friends, coworkers, and loved ones. The sense of "nothing else matters" can sap your self-regulation strength, making effective eating and exercising seem absolutely trivial during these difficult times.

Work or Financial Crises

Losing a job or suffering major financial problems can interfere substantially with weight control. These crises, like crises in personal relationships, can make weight control seem unimportant by comparison. I've heard many clients say, "How can I worry about the number of fat grams I eat when my world is crumbling around me?" Considerable self-regulatory resources must now get diverted into networking, consolidating resources, and rethinking careers.

Major Changes in Eating Environments

The following two stories show how major changes in environments can affect your eating patterns dramatically:

Arnie: "I got promoted a few months ago. I was really excited. It was a great opportunity. Unfortunately, it involved traveling two to three days per week. I figured, 'No big deal, I can handle this.' I didn't realize how much traveling around the country disrupted my usual routines. I found myself frustrated and irritated more of the time. Relaxation and cooling down time became less and less. I felt tired in the morning and found it difficult to exercise at my usual time. I wound up in meetings in which all kinds of food (like muffins, doughnuts, pizza, cheese and crackers) were carted in during all hours of the day and night. My eating and exercising habits began to break down and I began gaining weight."

Jane: "I got a divorce last year. The time before the divorce was the real struggle (for about two years). The divorce was a tremendous relief for me. My weight was reasonably stable during the years before the divorce. I couldn't believe it, but I gained twenty pounds during this past year. It was such an adjustment. All of a sudden, for the first time in ten years, I was living by myself. I thought that would make it so much easier to control my food. I didn't realize that being in an unhappy relationship in some ways created fewer temptations for me than being alone. I found myself feeling lonely. Other times, I went out with friends to dinners and parties—far more often than I had in the last ten years. I was drinking more and eating bar food. I had more trouble sleeping and that made it harder to get up early and exercise. I guess that's what did it."

As discussed in earlier chapters, traveling creates many challenges for weight controllers. Any substantial modification in your living situation also creates problems to be solved. Moving out of your house and into a college dormitory or moving out of a dormitory into an apartment are transitions with which you are probably familiar. If you recall those transitions in your life, consider the impact they had on your eating and exercising. Have you ever heard of the "Freshman Fifteen"? Many college freshmen report gaining fifteen pounds when they move into a college dormitory for the first time. These weight gains, while not documented scientifically, may occur for some people because of the tremendous changes in their usual routines.

Poor Problem Solving

A recent study compared "maintainers" to "regainers." Maintainers were formerly overweight women who had lost at least twenty pounds and maintained that loss for at least two years. Regainers were overweight women who regained weight within two years of losing at least twenty pounds. Regainers used "escape-avoidance" methods of solving problems much more so than did maintainers. These methods included eating, drinking, smoking, sleeping, and wishing the problems would just go away. Regainers also failed to get as much support from others ("social support") as did the maintainers.

Abstinence Violation Effect (AVE)

Psychologists have identified a type of distortion in thinking that creates problems. The abstinence violation effect, or AVE, first involves making a commitment to "abstinence." Many people who change their habits (for example, people who quit smoking or drinking alcohol, as well as successful weight controllers) make a commitment to abstain forever from a certain pattern of eating or drinking. Weight controllers who do this may view themselves as "dieters."

What happens when a dieter eats a food that is not on the diet? For example, what happens when someone on a low-carb diet eats a piece of birthday cake? This dieter may view this initial lapse as a major conflict. The conflict might sound something like this in the mind of the dieter: *How can I be a dieter if I ate a piece of birthday cake?* One way some resolve this conflict is to abandon dieting. In other words, abstinence violation effects are relapses that occur to reduce the internal conflict created by lapses. When weight controllers commit to unrealistically stringent standards for eating or exercising, they set the stage for AVEs. Following this commitment, initial lapses can produce major conflicts. These internal conflicts can be resolved by launching a full-blown slump: *I can eat cake now because I am no longer a dieter.*

Slump Busters

Whether your slump was caused by an injury, scale phobia, a vacation, stinkin' thinkin', or something else, now what? The following suggestions require action! Insight alone won't do it. Regaining momentum requires some notable action that leads to an even more notable change in your life.

Revisit Your Wellspring Plan

When consistent exercisers stop exercising, even for one day, they get rather testy. When weight controllers in the *Wellspring Plan* find their usual routines of eating, exercising, and monitoring disrupted, they also get testy. These individuals rely on a certain approach to eating and exercising and observing themselves in order to feel comfortable. Disruptions become sources of annoyance, irritability, and dissatisfaction. This is the heart of the *Wellspring Plan*, defining successful weight controllers; it shows a very strong commitment to permanent weight control.

Some weight controllers become secretly happy when opportunities to stray from their usual patterns emerge. You may have noticed this in yourself or others. "Oh well, I was at a party and there was nothing else to eat—so I ate!" If you truly embrace the *Wellspring Plan*, you will hold yourself to a higher standard. You would find it unacceptable to deviate from your plans without dealing with those deviations as problems. This doesn't mean that you berate yourself unmercifully when problems develop. It does mean that you see deviations as problems and attempt to deal with them directly. Wouldn't it be great if successful weight control meant having a happy-go-lucky attitude and feeling free of the oppression that seems required for success? It just doesn't work that way. The biology of excess weight is simply too tenacious. It takes a certain level of control, focus, and intensity to manage it effectively.

Some of my clients who have lost a lot of weight and kept it off for years have lamented, "Now that I've lost all this weight, I expected to feel good about myself most of the time. But I don't. I still struggle with this every day." Sadly, this is the nature of the battle with the biology of excess weight. Most people do not view their own successes at weight control as joyous accomplishments. People who lose a lot of weight are typically less than thrilled about their new weight statuses. Usually, they want to lose another five, ten, twenty, or more pounds. Even if they find their new weights acceptable, they still have to work hard to maintain their focus. There may be a certain "joy in the discipline." Exercise can bring its own rewards, as can a sense of control about eating patterns. Nevertheless, the state in which many successful weight controllers find themselves feels more like "healthy obsession" than "joyous accomplishment."

Health Clubs

Many years ago health clubs were places for fanatics, weightlifters, grunters and groaners, and athletes. Now, they serve as social melting pots. They also provide many comforts and a very wide range of activities. Low-impact and no-impact aerobic classes, spinning classes, water aerobics activities, yoga, instruction in almost every indoor sport imaginable, and machines, machines, machines. These centers of physical activity can serve as effective slump busters, but only if you actually use the club you join! The novelty and diversity of activities in health clubs can sometimes motivate refocusing on healthy eating and exercising.

When selecting a health club, keep in mind their three most important qualities: location, location, location! You will find that you actually use your health club when you either live very near it or work near it. If you belong to a health club located close to your house, you may use it in the morning. Almost all of the thousands of weight controllers with whom I have worked over the last thirty-four years and who have succeeded at this difficult enterprise have exercised primarily in the morning. Morning exercise proves most reliable because it interferes less with your daily life. After all, in the morning, you have complete control of your schedule and you can exercise before getting showered and dressed for the day. Exercising at any other time of the day requires taking a second shower and interrupting activities. Yet another advantage of morning exercise concerns attitude. You may have noticed that you feel better during the day if you exercise first thing in the morning. For all of these reasons, consider choosing a health club near your home, if at all possible.

Personal Trainers

Many people use trainers to help motivate them. Working with a trainer can help you learn about different types of equipment. For example, if you decide to begin a weightlifting program, a trainer could provide important instruction on technique and help you set up an effective regimen. Trainers can also provide encouragement and support. Also, if you set up an appointment with a trainer—particularly if you prepay for that appointment—you will motivate yourself, increasing your chances of doing some constructive exercising that day.

Try to find trainers who have advanced degrees in physical education or who are certified as athletic trainers. The American College of Sports Medicine certifies trainers, though the world's largest certifiers of trainers is the American Council on Exercise (ACE). ACE Certified Trainers have passed a rigorous test demonstrating a detailed knowledge of physical exercise and conditioning principles. If you select a trainer who has an advanced degree in physical education and/or appropriate certification, you can feel more confident that the advice you get is grounded in science rather than hearsay. Unfortunately, personal trainers can cost between $10 and $100 per hour. Prices vary depending on standards used within the health club, training, and whether the trainers come to your house or you go to their facilities. If you are in a major slump, paying the price of weekly sessions with a personal trainer for a month or two may well be worth it.

Equipment

"I couldn't get myself focused until I bought a treadmill. It was a major expense (almost $2,000), but I get on that thing every day now. I really like it. I like having it in my house because of the flexibility and the reminder it provides. When I see it sitting there (which is very easy because it's huge), I know how important the *Wellspring Plan* is to me." These sentiments were expressed by one of my former clients. She had indeed gotten into a major slump and was very excited about the way her new treadmill helped her get out of it.

An equipment purchase can prove very motivating for the reasons this former client outlined. Having the equipment in your home makes it much easier to exercise. Many people who have weight problems are reluctant to go to health clubs. They find the looks and comments of other people disconcerting. Of course, overweight people have as much right to use facilities at health clubs as any other customers. Yet the feelings can be so strong for some people that overcoming them is very difficult. Some people also live in climates that make outdoor exercising such as walking or jogging particularly challenging. These challenges can be overcome with appropriate clothing. However, when it's minus ten degrees or when it's icy outside, you won't find even hardy souls merrily walking around outside.

Some very adequate exercycles are available for a few hundred dollars. More elaborate pieces of high-quality equipment carry much higher price tags. The best way to decide which piece of equipment makes the most sense for you is to go to a health club and try out the equipment. If you try out various pieces of equipment for several weeks, you will determine which kind is most comfortable for you and which you might use consistently.

Consumer Reports routinely evaluates exercise equipment for home use. Your local library includes copies of recent issues of *Consumer Reports*. The publisher of this magazine also prints books and maintains a convenient Web site that summarizes their findings. Before spending hundreds, perhaps thousands, of dollars consider studying the available evidence about which pieces of equipment work most effectively and reliably.

Radical Changes in Diet

Radical changes in eating plans can sometimes break slumps. They require concentration, but may serve as rallying points for change. Usually, radical dietary approaches suffer the same fate as all diets: they do not work for very long. But as a temporary step, making a major shift in your eating plan could spark important changes. You could, for example, try a vegetarian approach.

Medications

Joe, a very obviously overweight middle-aged man, went to see his doctor about the new "diet" medications.

"Doc, I've got to have those new meds that will get me to believe I just ate a turkey dinner."

"Well, Joe, I don't know about the turkey dinner part, but they could help you lose weight if you're willing to work at it."

"But, Doc, I thought those pills made you feel like you just ate a turkey dinner *and* that you really want to work at it."

"Sorry, Joe, to really want to work at it, you have to find that within yourself somewhere—not in your medicine cabinet."

Physicians began prescribing amphetamines (Benzedrine) more than fifty years ago to help people lose weight. Unfortunately, not only did Benzedrine reduce appetite, it is an addictive drug that produces a "high" that people crave. Thousands of people became addicted to Benzedrine in an attempt to lose weight. That drug and others like it can no longer be prescribed in the United States or England for weight control. Prescriptions for those drugs are carefully monitored by governmental agencies.

Before beginning a discussion of the different medications available on the market today, it is critical to emphasize that it only makes sense to take these medications if you are participating in a professionally conducted weight control program. Scientific research suggests that these medications produce few benefits unless weight controllers get help focusing on eating and exercising through a professional program while taking them.

Many physicians know the sad tales of people like Joe. They believe any drug prescribed for weight control may cause more harm than good. This view, while understandable, no longer fits the current scientific information about medications for weight control. Despite the bias against them, some modern medications can help people decrease their appetite and feel full sooner. These efforts can occur with virtually no risk for causing addictions. Does this sound too good to be true?

Medications that help control appetite also can produce such side effects as depression, irritability, dizziness, insomnia, and nausea. The best of the medications produce very few of these effects for most people. However, these effects, when they occur, can be quite annoying. Also, the research on these medications suggests that they work well while they are taken. However, soon after they are discontinued, even if they were taken for six months or one year, many regain all of the weight they lost. Also, these medications generally produce small amounts of weight loss.

Modern medications for weight control still have an important role to play. First, if you take these medications while participating in an active weight control program, they might really help you. I have seen this happen with many of my clients. Their weight losses slowed down or stopped for various reasons. After they began a course of drug treatment, their eating and exercising improved markedly. I have seen quite a few people use the medications, lose ten to twenty pounds, get off the medications and continue to lose weight.

The medication popularly known as "Fen-Phen" (Fenfluramine-Phentermine, sometimes known as Pondimin and Ionamin) was used for more than ten years several decades ago. A related medication that was rather close in its effects to Fenfluramine (Pondimin), Redux (Dex-Fenfluramine), was the first appetite control medication approved by the Food and Drug Administration (FDA) in twenty-three years. Some recent case studies and some very expensive lawsuits led the manufacturers of both Pondimin and Redux to discontinue their availability in the fall of 1997. The scientific basis for this action was minimal.

A newer medication, Meridia (Sibutramine), acts like Fen-Phen and is the best available appetite control medication. Medical monitoring by physicians who know these medications is necessary to maximize safety and effectiveness. Any drug can produce side effects, some rather troubling, and these medications are no exception.

Another medication (Orlistat, sometimes called Xenical) contains an enzyme that blocks the absorption of fat, at least the absorption of about one-third of the fat consumed. Some preliminary research suggests that at least some people respond favorably to taking this medication and lose modest amounts of weight. However, if you follow the principles in this book (for example, eating as little fat as possible), Orlistat would not prove helpful. In addition, most people will experience some notable and troublesome digestive problems associated with taking a medication that extracts fat from food (including flatulence, oily stools, and bloating). Successful weight controllers tend to find ways of eating low-fat foods and making that a permanent part of their lifestyles. Reliance on this medication for that purpose seems unlikely as an effective long-term strategy. On the other hand, you could occasionally use a medication like this if you do overeat on high-fat foods. If taken within an hour of the problematic food or meal, it could decrease the impact of eating high-fat foods.

If prescription medications for weight control can help some participants in professional programs, can over-the-counter drugs (such as Dexatrim and others) help anyone? Probably not. One of the two non-prescription drugs that are available in the United States, phenylpropanolamine (PPA), acts like a mild stimulant. PPA can produce some small weight losses, but the effects do not last long. PPA is found in most non-prescription "weight control" drugs. Benzocaine, the other approved non-prescription drug, is found in some over-the-counter "appetite" or "weight control" drugs. It supposedly numbs taste, smell, or other qualities of food. It does not work.

If you want to try medications for weight control, first join a professional program. Then discuss this possibility with your therapist from that program and consider only prescription medications—if you and your therapist view that option as worthwhile.

Self-Help Programs and Books

Joining a program such as Take Off Pounds Sensibly (TOPS—www.tops.org) or Weight Watchers (www.weightwatchers.com) could be quite an effective slump buster. These programs cost either nothing (TOPS) or relatively modest amounts of money (Weight Watchers). Every major city in the United States and many smaller towns have TOPS chapters (ten thousand-plus nationwide) and Weight Watchers groups that meet frequently. These approaches provide support for change and may help you refocus.

Many self-help books, video tapes, CDs, and Web sites can help you refocus. Materials are available on relaxation, eating, nutrition, depression, visualization, and other topics that may reawaken your commitment to effective weight control. Among the better weight control Web sites are www.calorieking.com, www.weightwatchers.com, and www.ediet.com.

Professional Help

Hospitals and medical centers sometimes offer programs, such as Optifast (see www.optifast.com), that often can do a better job of helping people lose weight than self-help materials or programs can. Look for professionally conducted programs focused on weight loss directed by psychologists with expertise in "cognitive-behavior therapy." Programs that provide help for unlimited periods of time (no less than one year) are especially worthy of consideration. Web searches and calls to local hospitals, colleges, and universities (psychology departments), may prove helpful. The following two national organizations have relevant listings of psychologists in virtually every area of the United States: Association for Behavioral and Cognitive Therapies (www.ABCT.org, (212) 647-1890) and American Psychological Association (www.apa-helpcenter.org, (202) 336-5500).

Consumer Reports recently reported on the largest survey ever conducted among people who had obtained professional help for psychological problems other than, or in addition to, weight loss. More than four thousand readers of that magazine answered twenty-six questions about mental health professionals, family doctors, and support groups they sought for help with psychological distress. Among their most intriguing—and hopeful—findings were:

- People who obtain help from their family doctors tended to feel better after obtaining the help. But people who saw a mental health specialist for more than six months did much better.
- Most people who took medications for psychological problems (like Prozac) reported feeling better, but about half of the re-

spondents reported substantial and troublesome side effects (like drowsiness and a feeling of disorientation).

- The longer people stayed in therapy, the more they improved.
- Most people who went to a self-help group (like Alcoholics Anonymous) were very satisfied with the experience and said they felt much better.
- Almost everyone who sought help experienced some relief, but people who started out feeling the worst reported the most progress.

DEPRESSION

Mental health professionals define depression as including at least five of the following problems for at least two weeks. At least one of the problems must be either (1) depressed mood, or (2) loss of interest in pleasure.

1. Depressed mood, most of the day, nearly every day.
2. Markedly less interest or pleasure in all, or almost all, activities most of the day, nearly every day.
3. Significant weight loss or weight gain when not dieting, or increase in appetite nearly every day.
4. Insomnia or hypersomnia (excess sleeping) nearly every day.
5. Excess physical movement or slowing down in physical movements, nearly every day.
6. Fatigue or loss of energy every day.
7. Feelings of worthlessness or excessive or inappropriate guilt, nearly every day.
8. Decreased ability to think or concentrate, or indecisiveness, nearly every day.
9. Recurrent thoughts of death (not just fear of dying), recurrent suicidal thoughts without a specific plan or suicide attempt or specific plan for committing suicide.

Many people experience significant depressions and other forms of psychological distress at some points in their lives. You can imagine how depression can interfere with successful weight control. When feeling depressed, people struggle to stay focused on almost anything in their lives, let alone something as difficult as the *Wellspring Plan*. I have heard many people say, "I just didn't care." This statement often accompanies significant lapses or slumps. Unfortunately, once again, your biology has no sympathy. If you feel lousy, for whatever reason, your biology will be more than happy to add excess pounds.

People try many things to get out of depression and other unpleasant psychological states. You can try talking to close friends, taking vacations, or changing something significant in your life. When all of your best efforts do not produce positive change, consider taking the next step. You can seek professional help for marital problems or problems with your moods, such as depression. You can ask close friends or relatives for referrals to licensed professionals in your area whom they know or have heard good things about. You can also call your local hospital or university and ask how to get professional assistance.

Most health insurance policies cover substantial amounts of the costs involved with such treatment. Most communities also provide relatively low-cost counseling. You can find these services by calling your church or synagogue or your local mental health association.

If at all possible, try to find a therapist who is licensed in your state and is either a psychologist, social worker, or psychiatrist. Psychologists receive five to eight years of training beyond a bachelor's degree. This training focuses on the scientific aspects of helping people change. Social workers receive one to three years of training beyond a bachelor's degree, focusing on how to form good relationships with people and to understand resources available in communities that can prove helpful. Psychiatrists receive a medical degree and then several years of training beyond that to help them specialize in how to help people with significant problems in their lives.

Psychiatrists are the only mental health professionals who prescribe the most medications. In some states and in the armed forces, specially trained psychologists can also prescribe medications. Unfortunately, mood altering medications are prescribed too frequently to weight controllers, especially by psychiatrists. However, this may not be an advantage as many psychiatrists prescribe medications too quickly. You could find yourself being treated with a powerful set of medications (with sometimes complicated side effects) while other less chemical methods can produce better outcomes. Therefore, I recommend seeing a licensed psychologist or social worker before seeing a psychiatrist. If medications seem like they would be helpful to you, these other licensed mental health professionals will certainly recommend that you get a consultation from a psychiatrist in order to use such treatments. I believe that if you can find a way of changing without using medications, you will achieve better results and feel better in the long run.

Many weight controllers who become depressed delay getting help. Certainly problems take a while to resolve on your own. You may ask friends or family for help. You may read about the problem and attempt to change yourself. These efforts are worthy of admiration and respect. If and when they do not produce positive outcomes, however, please take action quickly. Your biology acts very quickly to cause you trouble. A lapse can turn quickly into a slump. To avoid this downward spiral, *action* must become your middle name. Your biology does not allow you to stay in a slump very long without punishing you much more severely than the person who doesn't struggle with weight problems.

Sport psychologists provide very similar advice to elite athletes. When athletes struggle with emotional issues, their performances decline, just as your weight increases. Performance declines can rapidly become major slumps. Major slumps can ruin careers. Athletes and weight controllers must take action quickly to grapple with whatever problems face them. Quick actions on the part of athletes can end slumps. The same applies to you.

Epilogue

In 1958, obesity expert Albert Stunkard summarized research from the previous thirty years of scientific efforts to control obesity by saying:

> Most obese persons will not stay in treatment for obesity. Of those who stay in treatment, most will not lose weight and of those who do lose weight, most will regain it.

The principles in this book suggest much greater optimism about how to manage this very tricky problem. This book is based on science. That science provides you with hope if you follow these principles. You can lose weight and keep it off if you are willing to understand the evidence provided by science and stay in the struggle, no matter what. The research on people who use these principles in more recent years provides a clear basis for hope:

- Only 12% of people involved in the 1928 through 1958 research lost twenty pounds or more; now, approximately 50% of those in the best treatment programs lose twenty pounds or more.
- 90% of participants in professional programs that use very restricted calorie intake and professional counseling lose twenty

pounds or more and 50% lose forty pounds or more, compared with only 1% in the research conducted in the first half of the twentieth century.
- At the Wellspring Academy of California, America's first comprehensive boarding school for overweight teenagers, the construction of a nearly perfect world for weight controllers built on the principles of the *Wellspring Plan* led to the following results for the first semester:

- fifty-five pounds average weight loss
- 20 to 40% improvements in strength and fitness

The following famous prose poem, penned for a conference for insurance salespeople in 1932 by former president Calvin Coolidge, focuses on a central truth for weight controllers in the *Wellspring Plan*. At the heart of overcoming slumps and frustrations lies a powerful commitment to persist regardless of the obstacles from within and without—no matter what. I sincerely hope you nurture this most critical quality within yourself every day.

Persistence

Nothing in the world can take the place of persistence.
Talent will not;
nothing is more common than unsuccessful people with talent.
Genius will not;
unrewarded genius is almost a proverb.
Education will not;
the world is full of educated derelicts.
Persistence and determination alone are omnipotent.

—CALVIN COOLIDGE, 1932

The Wellspring Plan for Overweight Children and Teens: A Parents' Guide to Healthier, Happier Children

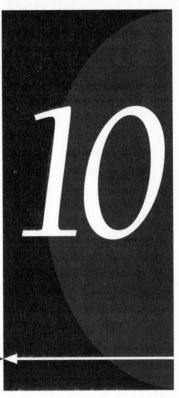

THE WORLD HEALTH ORGANIZATION recently declared that childhood obesity has officially become a worldwide epidemic. In the United States, about three times as many children and adolescents are obese today compared to 1980 (17% versus 5%). Overweight adolescents are at least ten times more likely to become obese adults than their non-overweight peers. This means that it will cost all Americans billions of dollars to care for the current generation of overweight youngsters as they age. Excess weight will cost these children even more than that. They are the ones who will suffer a wide variety of chronic medical maladies, social rejection, loss of productivity and opportunity at work, and emotional vulnerability. The purpose of this chapter is to describe, briefly, the causes of this epidemic, suggest a seven-step plan you can use to help your overweight child, and review the interventions currently available that help overweight children develop their own *Wellspring Plans*.

Obesogenic Environments: External and Internal Challenges

The past few decades have witnessed several cultural changes that make it almost natural for us to gain weight as we age. Think of your own lifestyle right now compared to people who lived in the 1950s and 1960s. You'll probably notice several things that make our current environments obesogenic (conducive to developing excess weight). Among them are:

- Very high-fat and sweet foods are more abundant and cheaper (in dollars adjusted for inflation). The increase in exportation of corn in the 1970s led to the development of high fructose corn syrup, a sweetener that is much cheaper and six times sweeter per gram than sugar. This has also improved the shelf life of bakery products and pastries in vending machines.
- More abundant food at cheaper prices has increased competition among food producers. Almost twice as many billions of dollars are spent now to market restaurants, soft drinks, and other problematic foods compared to the early 1980s.
- Marketing of high-sugar and high-fat foods has increasingly targeted children, including placement of vending machines and selling fast foods in thousands of elementary schools. These schools have grown dependent on the substantial profits available from such promotions, despite the unfortunate nutritional messages such products provide to young consumers.
- We're eating out 50% more than we did in 1975, including 50% more meals at fast food restaurants. These restaurants serve inexpensive but very high-fat foods.
- "Super-size me" has become a culturally understood phrase, as well as an award-winning documentary film. Portion sizes of fast foods and sugared drinks have doubled and tripled in the past few decades. The increased sizes make consumers feel they're getting more for their money and the restaurateurs certainly make far more profits on the super-sized foods. For example, it might cost the fast food company a penny to serve a one-quart "Big Gulp" for which many consumers happily pay an extra twenty-nine cents. That's a very tidy profit margin.

- We're far more sedentary than we used to be. Commutes in major cities have increased by 50% and the appeal of computers and home theaters equipped with electronic marvels has decreased movement among massive numbers of people. Children also spend far more time in structured and largely sedentary activities than they used to.
- As documented in the first chapter, even very intelligent weight controllers don't know what to do to regulate their weights because misinformation has been sold to them at alarming rates.

American culture clearly leans toward rapidly accelerating weight, a tragedy happening right now to millions of children and adolescents. Remember the major points made in Chapter 3 (*Know the Enemy—Your Biology*). The obesogenic external environment creates many challenges for everyone who wants to stay healthy and slim. The following biological realities, listed in Chapter 3, are relisted below to remind you what makes weight loss especially difficult for those with obesogenic internal environments:

- Genetics
- Fat Cell Number
- Fat Cell Size
- Insulin
- Lipoprotein Lipase
- Leptin
- Ghrelin
- Adiponectin
- Thermic Effect of Food
- Adaptive Thermogenesis
- Stomach Capacity
- Set-point

Fortunately, you can take some important steps to manage both external and internal challenges in your own home.

A Seven-Step Plan to Help Your Child Lose Weight

What do you do right now to help your overweight child? Perhaps you try to keep healthful foods well supplied. Maybe you model and encourage an active lifestyle. Let's consider seven steps that could take these actions and make them into an effective treatment for this extremely difficult and refractory problem:

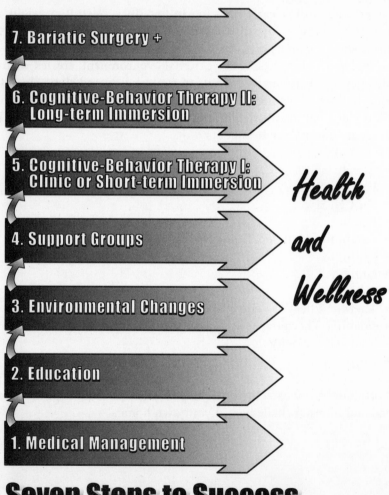

7. Bariatic Surgery +

6. Cognitive-Behavior Therapy II: Long-term Immersion

5. Cognitive-Behavior Therapy I: Clinic or Short-term Immersion

4. Support Groups

3. Environmental Changes

2. Education

1. Medical Management

Health and Wellness

Seven Steps to Success

Seven colleagues and I (a total of five physicians and three psychologists) created the seven steps approach pictured in the chart and published a paper about it in the February 2009 issue of the professional journal, *Obesity Management* (reprinted here with permission of the publisher, Mary Ann Liebert). The seven steps in the chart provide a roadmap. Each step has an arrow pointing to the ultimate goal of "Health and Wellness." That means that you can help your overweight child go directly from that step to achieve permanent weight control. Most families, however, find it necessary to add more intensive interventions (the steps with higher numbers) in order to succeed. Families that take these steps together achieve the best results.

Step 1. Medical Management. Seeing your child's pediatrician regularly will help provide you with feedback about progress and regular evaluations for potential health problems caused by excess weight (e.g., high blood pressure; liver problems; diabetes).

Steps 2 & 3. Education and Environmental Change. You could try to implement all eight steps of the *Wellspring Plan* as a family project. For example, everyone could self-monitor the day's eating and activities after dinner. Everyone could wear pedometers and agree to target ten thousand steps per day. You could even build in rewards, including money, contingent on your child's progress.

As you approach helping your child through this difficult process, it helps to review the suggestions made in Chapter 9 about supporting a family member's efforts to lose weight, reprinted here with modifications to apply to your child.

TABLE 10.1
HOW TO SUPPORT YOUR CHILD'S EFFORTS TO CONTROL HIS OR HER WEIGHT

Losing weight and keeping it off is a very difficult process. You can make it easier for your child. Here are several suggestions that will help you support and encourage weight controllers in your life:

General Attitude

Be positive. Convey to your child that even though it is very difficult to control weight, you believe he or she can do it. This attitude will boost his or her self-confidence while acknowledging the difficulties. Avoid negative comments, criticism, and coercion. These are unhelpful and demoralizing and will create negative feelings between you and your child. This, in turn, could cause him or her to eat more—not less—and thwart the likelihood of success in the long run.

Be reinforcing. Acknowledge your child's accomplishments. Compliments, attention, encouragement, and tangible reinforcement (like little gifts) can help him or her stay motivated and adhere to the plan.

TABLE 10.1 (CONTINUED)
HOW TO SUPPORT YOUR CHILD'S EFFORTS TO CONTROL HIS OR HER WEIGHT

General Attitude (continued)

Be realistic. Weight control requires tremendous effort and skill to overcome strong biological forces. People who are trying to lose weight must adopt eating and exercise patterns that are much more stringent than normal. Don't expect your child to be perfect, or even close to perfect. Occasional slips of overeating, inactivity, weight gain, and failure to adhere to plans will occur. Help your child learn from these experiences rather than dwell on them as "failures."

Communicate. If your child is a relatively independent teenager, occasionally inquire about his or her progress. Ask him or her how you can help, thereby complementing your teen's individual efforts. Be open to discussing the challenges of weight control and to assist in solving problems.

Managing Food

Increase the amount of nutritious, low-fat foods available to your child.

Do not encourage your child to eat foods that he or she is trying to avoid (for example, refrain from saying, "Let's go out for ice cream," or "Oh, come on, a little bit isn't going to hurt you").

Prepare food for your child in a low-fat way. Encourage experimentation and adventure.

Adopt appropriate eating habits, for example: not eating when full, eating appropriate portions, eating in a slow, deliberate fashion, eating regularly or on a schedule, limiting snacking, and limiting the number of eating situations. You may not have a weight problem, but better eating habits may improve your health and will support your child's efforts.

Plan activities with your child that do not revolve around food (for example, sporting events, concerts, games).

When you take your child to a restaurant, select places that make low-fat/low-sugar eating as pleasant as possible.

Promoting Exercise

Plan activities with your child that involve exercise (for example, walking, hiking, sports).

Exercise with your child. You will reap the same physical benefits.

Support and encourage your child's individual efforts to exercise.

Model an active lifestyle. This could involve becoming a more avid sports participant (e.g., tennis, golf), a regular health club user, using exercise equipment at home regularly, or just someone who seeks out, rather than avoids, movement. For example, when you have a choice about walking up a couple of flights of stairs rather than using an escalator, walk the stairs.

Use a pedometer yourself. Target ten thousand steps and consider posting your numbers and your child's numbers on a calendar on the refrigerator.

Create a reward system that reinforces monitoring of activity and achieving physical goals (like running a mile in less than nine minutes).

The primary addition to these suggestions concerns the importance of modeling the eating and activity patterns (see the last few bullet points above) you wish to encourage in your child. Following the dictum "do as I say, not as I do" is a prescription for failure for your child. You've got to walk the walk (literally in this case). That means eating healthful foods consistently and becoming a very active person. In addition, consider using the other tips below, all of which generally encourage you to model the *Wellspring Plan* behaviors and generously reinforce positive changes in your child.

Additional Tips to Help Your Child Change His or Her Eating and Activity Habits:

- Eliminate all high-fat foods in your home (remember, moderation doesn't work).
- Do not eat fattening foods in front of your child, ever.
- Encourage your child to take at least one bite of all food prepared. Have him or her rate the food from 0 (horrible) to 100 (the absolute greatest), and if the rating is very low, try preparing the food differently the next time or using different seasonings. For example, one of my sons actually likes broccoli, but only if he uses seasoned salt to flavor it.
- Have your child assist in shopping for and preparing healthful meals.
- Avoid using food as a reward.
- Try to limit TV and computer use to no more than two hours per day.
- Remove TVs and computers from your child's bedroom if at all possible.
- Establish a drink policy: Other than skim milk, only drink beverages with no calories (as noted in Step 3). These could include drinks with very few calories like Crystal Lite and Propel, but this rule excludes all fruit juices. Use one-a-day vitamins in pill form, not in juice form.

Step 4. Support Groups. Two well-known and widely available self-help groups have helped many people over the past fifty years. Take Off Pounds Sensibly has ten thousand groups in this country. Again, you can go to their Web site (www.tops.org) and click on "Chapter Locator" to find the location closest to your home. I did this and found the maximum number of chapters they list for searches like this (one hundred) within twenty-five miles of mine. Each chapter lists its meeting address and the name of chapter leaders with phone numbers. Many of these chapters welcome teenagers. TOPS focuses on self-monitoring and healthful eating and exercising, in a fashion consistent with the principles of the *Wellspring Plan*.

The only other nonprofessional approach that follows enough of the science of weight loss to warrant recommendation by this author is Weight Watchers. Weight Watchers also encourages healthful eating and self-monitoring and has over twenty thousand groups around the country (see www.weightwatchers.com). Their Web site lists locations for their groups with dates and times of the meetings. Some of them also welcome teenagers, although TOPS chapters seem more amenable in general to family involvement than do Weight Watchers.

The other nonprofessional approaches, like Overeaters Anonymous and Jenny Craig, have numerous flaws in their approaches from a scientific perspective.

Step 5. Cognitive Behavior Therapy (CBT) I: Clinic or Short-Term Immersion. CBT is a scientifically based approach to helping people improve their motivation, goal-setting, and focusing skills. Professionally conducted CBT programs for overweight children are available (check local hospitals, clinics). Immersion programs focus on CBT full time, for example for four weeks in the summer (e.g., www.wellspringcamps.com).

A weight loss camp could help your child considerably and efficiently (over four or eight concentrated weeks). You can find many weight loss camps with a few clicks of your mouse. What you will have a hard time finding are camps that take advantage of the opportunity to help make potentially permanent lifestyle changes based on science and relevant experience. The following factors help distinguish camps from each other and each is an important dimension for inclusion in the best camps:

American Camping Association Accreditation: The American Camping Association (ACA) is the premier organization that visits camps every three years to ensure that children across the country are attending camps that meet the minimum requirement for safe and enjoyable camping. The ACA standards are created by camp professionals and followed to ensure that ACA-accredited camps nationwide will offer safe and wonderful camping experiences.

Leadership: Leaders have credentials establishing expertise in education, educational management, clinical and scientific aspects of weight loss, behavioral psychology, and camping/outdoor education.

Clinical Program: Well-defined clinical intervention focused on intensive cognitive-behavior therapy conducted by appropriately trained and supervised staff.

Educational Program: Program clearly designed and staffed to increase knowledge of nutrition and psychological aspects of long-term weight control.

Diet: Low-Fat, Healthful, Balanced, Tasty, Fun: A food plan that focuses on very low-fat, but very enjoyable meals and snacks; the plan must exclude all high-fat foods and instead show variety and balance.

Diet: Uncontrolled Foods: Foods that are not portioned out or controlled are included in every meal.

Activities: An emphasis on a wide variety of activities, at least some of which could be maintained readily after camp; must include use of a pedometer to count steps in camp.

Family Involvement: Families are clearly involved in the change process (e.g., workshops; materials provided; staff available for consultation).

After-Care Program: Extensive post-camp intervention that includes sustained interactions with staff for at least three months.

Outcomes: Well-documented and clearly favorable outcomes using weight measures and additional measures (e.g., mood, self-esteem; parent and child ratings).

Location: Well located (e.g., beautiful setting, removed from city life).

Facilities: Comfortable and well maintained.

Insurance Reimbursement: Provision of a means to obtain reimbursement from health and/or medical insurance.

I serve as vice president, clinical services, for Wellspring Camps. As the table shows, the camps were designed in 2004 with the factors mentioned above very much in mind—122 campers attended two Wellspring Camps in 2004; more than 1,100 attended eleven Wellspring Camps and Wellspring Academy of California in the summer of 2010. The design of these camps was so unusual that they became the focus of many media stories, including a full-hour show on NBC's *Dateline* and a series of shows on both CNN and ABC's *20/20*. They have also been featured in stories that appeared in the *New York Times*, *Los Angeles Times*, *Washington Post*, and many other newspapers.

More important than the media coverage are the outcomes obtained by the campers, some of which were mentioned in previous chapters, showing rapid weight loss (almost four pounds per week) and addi-

	Wellspring Camps	Camp Shane	Camp Kingsmont	New Image Camps	Camp NuYu
American Camping Association Accreditation	✓			✓	
Leadership Expertise: Weight Loss, Psychology, Education, Camping	✓				
Clinical Program	✓		✓		
Educational Program	✓		✓		
Diet: Low-Fat, Healthful, Balanced, Tasty, Fun	✓				
Diet: Uncontrolled Foods	✓				
Activities: Lifestyle Emphasis	✓				✓
Family Involvement	✓				
After-Care Program	✓			✓	✓
Outcomes	✓				
Location	✓	✓	✓	✓	✓
Facilities	✓		✓	✓	✓
Insurance Reimbursement	✓				

Cost per week—about $1000. Some camps, those that provide cognitive-behavior therapy primarily, allow for some reimbursement via health insurance (averaging about $1000 of reimbursement).

tional significant weight loss even once the campers went home. The following chart makes another point about the outcomes, showing that the campers who self-monitored most consistently during camp were much more likely to lose additional weight once they went home. fifty-two percent of the most consistent self-monitors lost significant amounts of weight over the course of the six to nine-month follow-up evaluation; only 20% of the least consistent self-monitors lost weight during the follow-up period. These findings underscore the importance of self-monitoring specifically, and of the healthy obsession more generally, for successful weight control.

These results show that programs that immerse overweight children and teens in near-perfect weight-losing environments can really make a difference in their lives. Well-designed environments with supportive staff can help young weight controllers find the yellow brick road to a different life—and maybe even stay on it. The self-monitoring effects

CHART 10.1: SELF-MONITORING CONSISTENCY

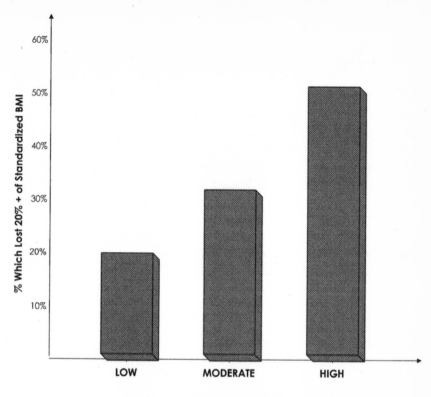

Consistency of Self-Monitoring During Camp

Wellspring Campers who self-monitored their eating and activities most consistently during camp were more likely to lose additional significant amounts of weight during the 6–9 month follow-up period.

show that a healthy obsession developed in camp can pay off down the road. These camps placed tremendous emphasis on the importance of self-monitoring, including creating rewards for consistent self-monitoring, providing reading materials and quizzes about its importance, and modeling of consistent self-monitoring by staff. The campers who were ready to accept these ideas and acted accordingly probably got closer to developing their own *Wellspring Plans* than those who weren't quite ready for this message.

Campers also improved their moods and self-esteem according to ratings that they provided and that their parents provided. It is possible that camps other than Wellspring Camps produce similar results, but published studies conducted on at least two camps didn't show effects as favorable as the ones seen at Wellspring.

Step 6. Cognitive Behavior Therapy II: Long-term Immersion. The only comprehensive boarding schools exclusively for overweight teens that exist in the United States today are the Wellspring Academies (see wellspringacademies.com). Wellspring's programs include many of the same elements as the best of the weight loss camps. As such, cognitive-behavior therapy is provided to facilitate change, and the diet and activity programs similarly provide substantial encouragement to move and to eat in accord with the *Wellspring Plan's* principles. The boarding school incorporates an academic program that allows students to keep up their schoolwork or make up work that they missed in schools at home. The long-term effects of this intensive model remain to be seen. However, the uniqueness of this approach has generated even more attention than Wellspring Camps (see wellspringweightloss. com, click on "In the News") and the initial outcomes are remarkable. Chart 10.2 shows the results comparing the findings from immersion programs (six studies) to outpatient programs to educational controls. These findings were summarized in two review papers, one published in 2010 and the other currently in press. Notice the huge difference in reduction in weight (in this case measured as percent overweight), with immersion treatments that use cognitive-behavior therapy (CBT) showing the best results by far.

Step 7. Bariatric Surgery +. For some seriously overweight teenagers who have tried the first six steps, specialized surgeries (bariatric surgeries like the gastric bypass) performed in surgical centers that have experience and understanding of this problem are important options (e.g., http://fitprogram.ucla.edu/). The "+" part of this step was included to emphasize the importance of choosing programs for these invasive and somewhat risky permanent procedures that include careful screening and good follow-up support programs.

CHART 10.2. IMMERSION TREATMENTS SHOW PROMISE FOR LONG-TERM
BENEFITS COMPARED TO OUTPATIENT PROGRAMS AND EDUCATIONAL
CONTROLS

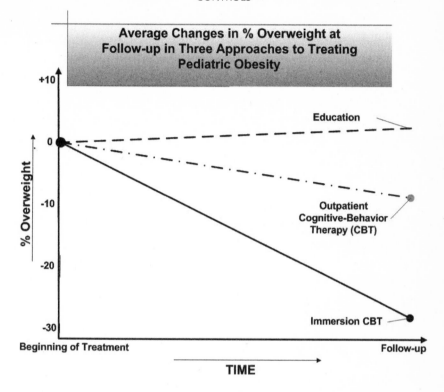

Summary and Conclusions

The seven steps presented in this chapter encourage you to keep add-ing levels of structure if needed to help your overweight child develop his or her own *Wellspring Plan*. The more aggressive interventions in Steps 5 through 7 may well become important options if the simpler earlier steps do not produce the desired results. The central theme here is to stay persistent and aggressive in efforts to change the entire family's approach to a healthful lifestyle. "Do as I say, not as I do" doesn't work. You've got to get involved and live the *Wellspring Plan* yourself in order for your child to make the transition from overweight to health-oriented and healthy.

Recipes from Wellspring Chefs

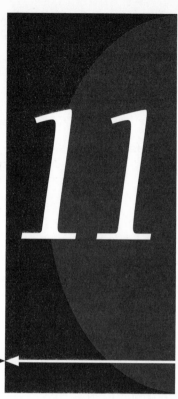

11

THE FIFTY-PLUS WONDERFUL RECIPES in this chapter were developed by myself and the chefs and food service staff from Wellspring. As such, these recipes yield very lovable foods that contain minimal fat, considerable fiber, and plant protein instead of animal protein in many cases. Hundreds of adolescents and staff members have tested these recipes and enjoyed them—and in some cases made suggestions to improve upon their predecessors.

Many of these recipes take very little effort to prepare and yield big dividends in taste and nutritional value. We hope you'll try these, experiment with variations on them, and pass them along to your friends.

BREAKFAST

Crêpes

DAVID BURNS

INGREDIENTS:
½ cup skim milk
½ cup water
¾ cup flour
2 ounces (¼ cup) Egg Beaters
1½ teaspoons vegetable oil

METHOD:
1. Combine all ingredients into a bowl and mix until smooth.
2. Allow to rest for 20 minutes.
3. To make each crêpe, ladle 2 tablespoons of the batter into a crêpe pan, cook on the first side until the edges look dry.
4. Turn the crêpe once and cook briefly on the second side.

YIELD:
12 crêpes, 6 servings of 2 each

NUTRITIONAL INFORMATION:
Calories 75
Protein........... 3 grams
Fat .... 1.3 grams
Carbs .... 12 grams

Strawberry Blintzes

DAVID BURNS

INGREDIENTS:

12 ounces fat-free cream cheese
¼ cup skim milk
½ teaspoon almond extract
12 crêpes (see previous recipe)
24 ounces strawberries, fresh

METHOD:

1. Preheat oven to 250 degrees.
2. Soften cream cheese in a microwave oven (30 seconds on high).
3. Combine cream cheese, skim milk and almond extract. Mix well.
4. Place one ounce (two tablespoons) of cream cheese mixture in each crêpe.
5. Roll crêpes and place on a 2-inch baking dish.
6. Top with 2 ounces of fresh strawberries.
7. Place crêpes in oven and warm for 15 minutes.

YIELD:

12 crêpes, 6 servings, 2 crepes per serving

NUTRITIONAL INFORMATION:

Calories 100
Protein........... 4.3 grams
Fat. .... 5 grams
Carbs .... 5 grams

Potato Pancakes

DAVID BURNS

INGREDIENTS:

2½ pounds potatoes
4 ounces (½ cup) onions, chopped
2½ ounces (¼ cup plus one tablespoon) Egg Beaters
6 tablespoons flour
½ teaspoon salt
¼ teaspoon baking powder
⅛ cup skim milk

METHOD:

1. Peel and shred potatoes.
2. In a mixing bowl combine potatoes, onion, egg substitute, flour, salt, baking powder and skim milk.

3. Heat griddle or frying pan to 350 degrees.
4. Pour ¼ cup of mixture onto griddle and turn after 3 to 4 minutes, or until golden brown.
5. Heat the second side, and then remove from griddle.

YIELD: 16 pancakes, 8 servings, 2 pancakes per serving

NUTRITIONAL INFORMATION:
Calories 114
Protein........... 4.5 grams
Fat .... 0 grams
Carbs .... 23 grams

French Toast

MEGAN O'REILLY

INGREDIENTS:
4 tablespoons egg whites
2 teaspoons skim milk
Dash of vanilla
4 pieces of multigrain or similar whole grain bread
Dash of nutmeg

METHOD:
1. Mix egg whites, skim milk, vanilla and nutmeg in a shallow bowl.
2. Lightly spray skillet with nonfat spray and heat on stovetop at medium heat.
3. When skillet is ready, lay bread slices in bowl one at a time so that each side is coated with mixture. Place slice in skillet.
4. Turn bread over after a few minutes (as soon as toast is browned) and heat second side until it is browned.
5. Serve with maple syrup and fat-free vanilla yogurt.

YIELD: 2 servings (2 slices each)

NUTRITIONAL INFORMATION:
Calories 164
Protein........... 4 grams
Fat .... 2 grams
Carbs .... 32.5 grams

Spotted Dog

MEGAN O'REILLY

INGREDIENTS:

1 cup brown rice
¼ cup raisins
¼ teaspoon cinnamon
1 tablespoon brown sugar
2 tablespoons skim milk

METHOD:

1. Mix rice, raisins, cinnamon and sugar in a medium bowl.
2. Bring 2 cups of water to a boil then add rice mixture to water.
3. Return to boil and simmer for 20 minutes or until most of the water is evaporated.
4. Add milk (more if a creamier mixture is desired).

YIELD:

4 servings (1 cup each)

NUTRITIONAL INFORMATION:

Calories .... 225 calories
Protein........... 9 grams
Fat .... 1.5 grams
Carbs .... 43.9 grams

Frittata

MEGAN O'REILLY

INGREDIENTS:

2 cups chopped onion
3 cups chopped broccoli
1 sliced large white mushroom or 2-3 small Portobello mushrooms
Dash of thyme
¾ teaspoon black pepper
3 cups egg whites
1 cup fat-free Mozzarella cheese

METHOD:

1. Preheat oven to 350 degrees.
2. Lightly spray nonfat cooking spray in a skillet and heat on stove on medium.
3. Sauté onions until clear.
4. Add broccoli and continue to sauté for 4 to 5 minutes; add mushrooms and cook until soft.
5. Sprinkle with thyme and black pepper.

6. Reduce heat to medium-low and pour egg over vegetables.
7. Turn heat to low and continue to heat.
8. As eggs solidify sprinkle cheese on top.
9. Heat on stovetop until edges begin to firm.
10. Heat in oven for 5 to 10 minutes or until center is firm.

YIELD: 8 servings (1 cup each)

NUTRITIONAL INFORMATION: Calories 94
                                Protein .... 18 grams
                                Fat .... 0 grams
                                Carbs .... 5.5 grams

LUNCH

PIZZA AND PIZZA-STYLE RECIPES

Basic Pizza Crust
DAVID BURNS

INGREDIENTS: ⅔ cup warm water
                                1¾ cups flour
                                1 teaspoon sugar
                                1 teaspoon yeast
                                ½ teaspoon salt

METHOD: 1. In a mixing bowl combine water, flour, sugar, yeast and salt.
                                2. Knead with a dough hook at medium speed or by hand until a smooth, elastic dough forms (about 10 minutes).
                                3. Place the dough in a warm area and cover with a warm, damp towel. Allow the dough to rise until it doubles in size.
                                4. Turn the dough out on a lightly floured cutting board and release the air in the dough by kneading briefly. Shape the dough into 6 small balls and allow proofing a second time (about an hour).
                                5. Flatten each dough ball into a 7-inch wide

circle, add toppings as desired and bake in a 550-degree oven for about 10 minutes or until golden brown and crisp.

ALTERNATIVE USES:

1. **Pita Bread:** Follow steps 1 through 6 but do not add toppings. Bake about 13 minutes in a 550-degree oven. When removed from the oven, the bread deflates and a pocket forms.
2. **Grilled bread or Boboli style:** Prepare the basic pizza dough but grill the bread 3 to 4 minutes on each side until the bread blisters, puffs and cooks through.

YIELD:

6 servings (3 ounces each)

NUTRITIONAL INFORMATION:
(WITHOUT TOPPINGS)

Calories 134
Protein........... 4 grams
Fat .... 0.4 grams
Carbs .... 28 grams

Basic Cheese Pizza
DAVID BURNS

INGREDIENTS:

Six 7-inch pizza crusts
1 cup pizza sauce
8 ounces light shredded mozzarella cheese
2 ounces shredded Parmesan cheese

METHOD:

1. Preheat oven to 550 degrees.
2. Prepare basic pizza crust as directed.
3. Spread enough pizza sauce to cover each crust.
4. Top with enough mozzarella and Parmesan cheese to lightly coat each crust.
5. Bake in oven for about ten minutes or until crust is slightly brown and cheese is melted.

YIELD:

6 servings

NUTRITIONAL INFORMATION:
(EXCLUDING THE CRUST)

Calories 103
Protein........... 7.9 grams
Fat .... 3.3 grams
Carbs .... 9.1 grams

Pita Pocket Pizza
DAVID BURNS

INGREDIENTS:
6 pita pockets
12 ounces (1½ cups) pizza sauce
6 ounces fat-free shredded Jack cheese
6 ounces fat-free shredded cheddar cheese

METHOD:
1. Preheat oven to 350 degrees.
2. Place pita pockets on a clean surface.
3. Spread 2 ounces of pizza sauce on each pocket.
4. Top each with 1 ounce of Jack cheese and 1 ounce of cheddar cheese.
5. Sprinkle cheese with water.
6. Bake in oven for 10 to 15 minutes or until cheese is thoroughly melted.

YIELD:
6 servings

NUTRITIONAL INFORMATION:
Calories 260
Protein .... 25 grams
Fat .... 0 grams
Carbs .... 40 grams

Pizza Mexicana
DAVID BURNS

INGREDIENTS:
4 fat-free 6-inch flour soft taco tortillas
8 ounces (half a 16-ounce can) fat-free refried beans
3 fresh tomatoes, diced
8 ounces fat-free shredded Jack cheese

METHOD:
1. Preheat oven to 350 degrees.
2. Place tortillas on a cookie sheet.
3. Spread 2 ounces of the refried beans on each tortilla.
4. Spread the tomatoes on top of the refried beans.
5. Top each pizza with 2 ounces of cheese.
6. Sprinkle cheese with a small amount of water.
7. Bake in oven until cheese melts.

YIELD:
4 servings

NUTRITIONAL INFORMATION:
Calories 232
Fat .... 0.18 grams
Protein........... 23.5 grams
Carbs............. 35 grams

Grilled Mandarin Chicken Pita Sandwich
RYAN OSTRANDER

INGREDIENTS:
1 pound boneless, skinless chicken breasts
2 tablespoons low-calorie, no-oil Italian dressing
1 teaspoon soy sauce
2 tablespoons chopped chives
2 cups chopped romaine lettuce
2 cups mandarin oranges (canned in water)
4 whole wheat pitas

METHOD:
1. Preheat grill to 350 degrees.
2. Grill chicken breasts until done then place in refrigerator to cool.
3. In a large bowl, combine Italian dressing, soy sauce and chives and set aside.
4. Cut grilled chicken breasts in cubes and add to dressing. Let marinate for 30 minutes.
5. After marinated, add full contents of chicken mixture to romaine and mandarin oranges in a bowl and toss until evenly coated.
6. Cut pita into halves and open them into pockets.
7. Add lettuce mixture to pockets and serve.

YIELD:
4 servings (1 stuffed pita each)

NUTRITIONAL INFORMATION:
Calories 310.25
Protein........... 29.45 grams
Fat .... 2.9 grams
Carbs............. 41.6 grams

Teriyaki Rice Bowl

DAVID BURNS

INGREDIENTS:
½ cup teriyaki marinade
1 pound boneless, skinless chicken breasts
4 ounces (½ cup) chopped green onions
2 cups cooked long grain rice

METHOD:
1. In a large bowl pour ½ cup of teriyaki marinade.
2. Coarsely chop chicken breasts into 1-inch by ½-inch pieces.
3. Add chicken and onions to marinade. Marinate for 45 minutes.
4. Heat stovetop to medium-high and lightly spray a skillet with nonfat cooking spray.
5. Remove chicken and onions from marinade and quickly grill until done.
6. Place 5-ounce serving of chicken and onions over ½ cup cooked rice.

YIELD:
4 servings (9 ounces each)

NUTRITIONAL INFORMATION:
Calories 289
Protein .... 36.63 grams
Fat .... 4 grams
Carbs .... 26 grams

Vegetarian Lasagna

JACQUELYN WINDFELDT

INGREDIENTS:
1 package (10 ounces) of lasagna noodles
32 ounces fat-free ricotta cheese (32 ounces fat-free cottage cheese may be substituted, but must be drained)
⅔ cup Egg Beaters, or egg whites
3 green onions, diced
2 cups pre-made pasta sauce
1 medium-sized yellow/red/green pepper, chopped
1 bag (10 ounces) frozen spinach, thawed
2 cups fat-free mozzarella cheese
½ cup fat-free Parmesan cheese

METHOD:
1. Preheat oven to 350 degrees.
2. Cook lasagna noodles according to the

instructions on package or until noodles are firm.

3. Mix peppers, spinach and onions together.
4. Mix vegetable mixture, ricotta cheese, egg substitute and onions in a medium bowl.
5. In a 12-inch by 14-inch baking pan, layer cooked noodles, ricotta mixture and sauce and repeat until all is used. Add in up to half of the mozzarella.
6. Top layers with remaining mozzarella and Parmesan cheese.
7. Cover pan with a sheet of aluminum foil and bake lasagna for 1 hour (remove foil for the last 15 minutes so that top layer is slightly browned).

YIELD: 12 servings (6 ounces/ ¾ cup each)

NUTRITIONAL INFORMATION:
Calories 156
Protein........... 12 grams
Fat .... 0.6 grams
Carbs .... 25.6 grams

DINNER

Buffalo Stew
DAVID BURNS

INGREDIENTS:
2 pounds buffalo stew meat in 1-inch cubes*
½ gallon water
1½ teaspoon Worcestershire sauce
2 cloves garlic
1½ teaspoon paprika
2 pounds red potatoes, quartered
2 stalks celery, chopped
1 pound carrots, chopped
8 ounces (1 cup) onions, chopped
Cornstarch (optional)
Beef broth to taste (small amount)

METHOD:
1. In a large stew pot, brown the buffalo meat on high heat (about 3 minutes).

2. Add water, Worcestershire sauce, garlic and paprika.
3. Cover and cook on low heat for 3 hours.
4. Add vegetables and cook for an additional 30 minutes.
5. Adjust flavor and color by adding beef broth to taste.
6. For a thicker sauce add cornstarch until attaining desired texture.

YIELD: 6 servings (12 ounces each)

NUTRITIONAL INFORMATION:
Calories 204
Protein........... 9 grams
Fat .... 1.87 grams
Carbs .... 37.5 grams

*NOTE: Go to buffalogal.com or buffaloguys.com to order buffalo or ask your local grocer to order some for you.

Buffalo Meatloaf
DAVID BURNS

INGREDIENTS:
1½ pounds ground buffalo
2 slices bread, crumbled
½ cup skim milk
2½ ounces (¼ cup plus one tablespoon) Egg Beaters
1 ounce (⅛ cup) onion, chopped
1½ teaspoons table salt
1½ teaspoons pepper

METHOD:
1. Preheat oven to 325 degrees.
2. Combine all ingredients in a mixing bowl and beat at low speed until blended.
3. Pour ingredients into a small loaf pan.
4. Bake at 325 degrees for 1½ hours.

YIELD: 6 servings (6 ounces each)

NUTRITIONAL INFORMATION:
Calories 160
Protein........... 26 grams
Fat .... 2.12 grams
Carbs .... 9.25 grams

Ginger Pineapple Chicken Stir-Fry with Snow Peas

RYAN OSTRANDER

INGREDIENTS:

1 tablespoon sesame seeds
1 tablespoon chopped garlic
1 pound boneless, skinless chicken breasts, cut into 2-inch strips
1 red bell pepper cut into strips
1 red onion, roughly chopped
1 tablespoon minced fresh ginger
¾ cup sliced shiitake mushrooms
½ cup soy sauce
1 cup fresh pineapple chunks
1 teaspoon red pepper flakes
2 cups fresh snow peas

METHOD:

1. Spray nonstick frying pan with a nonfat cooking spray. Add sesame seeds, chopped garlic and chicken strips to the pan and sauté for 2 minutes.
2. Add red pepper, onion, ginger and mushrooms. Continue to sauté for 1 minute.
3. Add soy sauce, pineapple, red pepper flakes and snow peas. Cover and let cook for 1 minute.
4. Uncover and stir until chicken and vegetables are covered with sauce and chicken is fully cooked.

YIELD:

4 servings (8 ounces each)

NUTRITIONAL INFORMATION:

Calories 243
Protein .... 29.93 grams
Fat .... 3.68 grams
Carbs .... 22.5 grams

Roasted Cod Fillet with Blueberry & Black Cherry Salsa

RYAN OSTRANDER

INGREDIENTS:

1 tablespoon granulated sugar
½ cup raspberry vinegar
1 pint fresh blueberries
1 pint black cherries, quartered with pits removed
2 tablespoons diced red onion
1 medium-sized yellow tomato, diced
1 medium-sized orange bell pepper, diced
¼ cup freshly chopped basil
½ teaspoon salt
¼ teaspoon black pepper
4 Atlantic cod fillets (about 4 ounces each)
4 slices of lemon
¼ teaspoon freshly chopped garlic

METHOD:

1. To make salsa, combine sugar and vinegar in a bowl and whisk until sugar is dissolved. In a separate bowl stir together blueberries, black cherries, red onion, yellow tomato, orange pepper, basil, garlic, salt and black pepper. Add sweetened vinegar to bowl and allow to marinate for 30 minutes.
2. Next, preheat oven to 400 degrees. Arrange fish on a nonstick baking sheet and place a slice of lemon on each fillet. Roast for 12 to 15 minutes or until done.
3. Remove lemon slices, top with salsa and serve.

YIELD: 4 servings (6 ounces each)

NUTRITIONAL INFORMATION:
Calories 190
Protein .... 21.23 grams
Fat .... 1.75 grams
Carbs .... 22.3 grams

Sour Cream Chicken

DAVID BURNS

INGREDIENTS:

1¼ pounds boneless, skinless chicken breasts
2 cups fat-free chicken broth
5 tablespoons paprika
½ teaspoon salt
2 cups fat-free sour cream
2 teaspoons flour

METHOD:

1. Preheat oven to 350 degrees and lightly spray a pan or oven-safe dish with nonfat cooking spray.
2. Place chicken breasts in pan and bake for 20 minutes. Set aside.
3. Spray a skillet with nonfat cooking spray. Add onions and sauté until translucent, not brown.
4. Add chicken broth, paprika and salt and reduce heat to low.
5. In a separate bowl, mix together the sour cream and flour.
6. Slowly add sour cream mixture to the broth and mix well.
7. Add reserved chicken breasts and simmer until chicken is heated through and the sauce has thickened.

YIELD:

5 servings (4 ounces each)

NUTRITIONAL INFORMATION:

Calories 201
Protein .... 31 grams
Fat .... 1.66 grams
Carbs .... 15.5 grams

Chicken Nuggets

DAVID BURNS

INGREDIENTS:

12 ounces boneless, skinless chicken breasts
1 cup cornflakes
1 teaspoon paprika
½ teaspoon Italian herb seasoning
1 teaspoon garlic powder
¼ teaspoon onion powder
½ teaspoon salt

METHOD:

1. Preheat oven to 400 degrees and lightly spray a cooking sheet with nonfat spray.
2. Cut chicken breasts into bite-sized pieces.
3. Place cornflakes in plastic bag and crush with a rolling pin.
4. Add remaining ingredients to crushed cornflakes. Close bag and shake until blended.
5. Add a few chicken pieces at a time to the crumb mixture. Shake well to coat evenly.
6. Place chicken pieces on cooking sheet so they are not touching.
7. Bake for 12 to 14 minutes, or until golden brown.

YIELD:

4 servings

NUTRITIONAL INFORMATION:

Calories 168
Protein........... 27 grams
Fat .... 3.13 grams
Carbs .... 7.75 grams

Teriyaki Chicken Kabobs

DAVID BURNS

INGREDIENTS:

½ cup teriyaki marinade
1 pound boneless, skinless chicken breasts
1 green bell pepper
1 red bell pepper
8 medium-sized mushrooms
1 red onion
8 cherry tomatoes

METHOD:

1. Soak 4 8-inch metal skewers in water.
2. Cut chicken breasts into 1-ounce portions.

3. Cut bell peppers and onions into 1-inch squares.
4. Pour the marinade into a large bowl and add in the chicken and vegetables. Marinate for 45 minutes.
5. Preheat oven to 350 degrees.
6. Build kabobs by stringing chicken and vegetables onto the skewer. Each skewer should contain 4 pieces of chicken.
7. Place kabobs on a cooking sheet and spray with nonfat cooking spray.
8. Bake for 20 minutes or until chicken is done.

YIELD: 4 kabobs

NUTRITIONAL INFORMATION (PER KABOB)

Calories 236
Protein .... 33 grams
Fat .... 4.3 grams
Carbs .... 16.3 grams

SALADS

Croutons

DAVID BURNS

INGREDIENTS:

4 slices French bread
6 ounces fat-free beef broth

METHOD:

1. Preheat oven to 275 degrees.
2. Soak the bread in beef broth and place on cookie sheet lined with parchment paper.
3. Slowly dry bread in oven for 30 minutes.
4. Flip the bread and continue drying until croutons are crisp and brown, about 30 minutes more.
5. Allow to cool and cut to desired size.

YIELD: 4 servings (1 ounce each)

NUTRITIONAL INFORMATION:

Calories 20
Protein .... 1 gram
Fat .... 0 grams
Carbs .... 4 grams

Fat-Free Thousand Island Dressing
DAVID BURNS

INGREDIENTS:

3 tablespoons chili sauce
1 tablespoon sweet pickle relish
8 ounces (1 cup) fat-free mayonnaise

METHOD:

1. Combine ingredients in a small mixing bowl.
2. Cover and chill for 60 minutes.

YIELD:

5 servings (1 ounce each)

NUTRITIONAL INFORMATION:

Calories 23
Protein .... 0.9 grams
Fat .... 0 grams
Carbs .... 4.88 grams

Tuna Salad
DAVID BURNS

INGREDIENTS:

8 ounces tuna, canned in water, drained
2½ ounces (¼ cup) fat-free mayonnaise
1 teaspoon sweet pickle relish

METHOD:

1. Combine all ingredients in a mixing bowl.
2. Chill for 45 minutes.

YIELD:

4 servings

NUTRITIONAL INFORMATION:

Calories 58
Protein .... 10 grams
Fat .... 0.37 grams
Carbs .... 2 grams

Egg Salad
DAVID BURNS

INGREDIENTS:

8 ounces (1 cup) Egg Beaters
2 ounces (¼ cup) fat-free mayonnaise
⅛ teaspoon white pepper
½ teaspoon red wine vinegar

METHOD:

1. Scramble Egg Beaters according to package directions.
2. Cool eggs for 30 minutes.

3. In a large bowl, combine the Egg Beaters with the remaining ingredients.

YIELD: 5 servings (2 ounces each)

NUTRITIONAL INFORMATION: Calories 30
Protein .... 4 grams
Fat .... 0.06 grams
Carbs .... 2.75 grams

Chinese Chicken Salad

DAVID BURNS

INGREDIENTS:
12 ounces boneless, skinless chicken breasts
10 ounces iceberg lettuce, shredded
4 ounces (6 teaspoons) fresh cilantro
8 green onions, sliced
1½ ounces cellophane rice noodles
2 tablespoons Kikkoman fat-free Chinese chicken salad dressing

METHOD:
1. Roast or boil chicken breasts until done. Allow to cool.
2. Toss iceberg, cilantro and green onions.
3. Cut chicken breasts into strips.
4. Place 3 ounces of lettuce mix on each of four plates.
5. Top each with 3 ounces of chicken breast.
6. Garnish with cellophane noodles.
7. Drizzle 2 tablespoons of salad dressing over chicken.

YIELD: 4 servings

NUTRITIONAL INFORMATION: Calories 239
Protein .... 28 grams
Fat .... 1.7 grams
Carbs .... 12 grams

Shrimp Louie
DAVID BURNS

INGREDIENTS:

12 ounces cooked shrimp
8 ounces iceberg lettuce, chopped
8 cherry tomatoes
2 ounces asparagus, canned and drained
4 stalks celery, cut into 1-inch slices
8 tablespoons fat-free Thousand Island dressing
(see recipe on p. 276)

METHOD:

1. Place cooked shrimp in a colander and rinse thoroughly.
2. Spread 2 ounces of chopped lettuce on each of four dinner plates.
3. Place 3 ounces of shrimp on top of lettuce.
4. Top with cherry tomatoes, asparagus, celery and a drizzle of 1 ounce of dressing.

YIELD:

4 servings (4 ounces each)

NUTRITIONAL INFORMATION:

Calories 191
Protein .... 19 grams
Fat .... 1.8 grams
Carbs .... 24.5 grams

Grilled Asparagus and Sweet Pepper Salad
RYAN OSTRANDER

INGREDIENTS:

1 pound fresh asparagus spears
1 medium-sized orange bell pepper
1 small or medium-sized red onion
1 lemon
1 lime
1 orange
¼ cup vinegar
2 tablespoons Dijon mustard

METHOD:

1. Preheat grill to 375 degrees.
2. Prepare vegetables for grilling by trimming off rough ends of asparagus, cutting the pepper in half and removing the seeds and slicing the onion.
3. Grill asparagus for only 2 or 3 minutes (you still want it crunchy). Continue grilling the onion and the pepper until they are flavored

but still crunchy. Place in refrigerator to cool down.
4. Zest the lemon, lime and orange and set aside.
5. Squeeze juice from the lemon, lime and orange and set aside.
6. In a large bowl, combine vinegar, Dijon mustard, salt, pepper and citrus juices.
7. Chop the onion and pepper and cut the asparagus into thirds.
8. Add the citrus zest and vegetables to the Dijon vinaigrette and toss until evenly coated.

YIELD: 4 servings (6 ounces each)

NUTRITIONAL INFORMATION:
Calories 64.25
Protein .... 3.18 grams
Fat .... 0.78 grams
Carbs .... 11.13 grams

Shrimp Cocktail
DAVID BURNS

INGREDIENTS:
1 pound shrimp, cooked and peeled
¾ cup ketchup
1 lemon, juiced
1 teaspoon Worcestershire sauce
1 teaspoon horseradish

METHOD:
1. Rinse and drain shrimp.
2. In a small mixing bowl combine ketchup, lemon juice, Worcestershire sauce and horseradish.
3. Transfer cocktail sauce into a supreme bowl or other appropriate container.
4. Arrange shrimp on a platter or other appropriate serving container.
5. Garnish with celery sticks and/or lemon wedges.

YIELD: 5 servings (4 ounces each)

NUTRITIONAL INFORMATION:
Calories 87
Protein .... 12.1 grams
Fat .... 1.19 grams
Carbs .... 6.98 grams

SOUPS

═══════════════

Split Pea Soup (An AOS Favorite)
DAVID BURNS

INGREDIENTS:
½ gallon water
1 cup dry split peas
2 stalks celery, finely chopped
½ onion, diced
4 ounces (½ cup) diced carrots
2 cloves garlic, minced
Salt to taste
Pepper to taste

METHOD:
1. Pour water into a large pot.
2. Add peas, celery, onion, carrots and garlic.
3. Bring entire mixture to a boil; simmer for one hour.
4. Add salt and pepper to taste.

YIELD:
8 servings (8 ounces each)

NUTRITIONAL INFORMATION:
Calories 61.75
Protein .... 5.6 grams
Fat .... 0.01 grams
Carbs .... 9.8 grams

Strawberry Cantaloupe Soup
RYAN OSTRANDER

INGREDIENTS:
1 medium-sized cantaloupe, peeled and cut into chunks
1 pint strawberries, stems removed
1 cup skim milk
1 cup fat-free plain yogurt
¼ cup granulated sugar
1 teaspoon vanilla extract
½ teaspoon ground cinnamon
1 tablespoon freshly chopped mint

METHOD:
1. In a blender or food processor add cantaloupe, strawberries, skim milk, fat-free yogurt, sugar and vanilla.

2. Blend on medium-high for about 2 minutes or until consistency is smooth.
3. Remove soup from blender or processor and pour into a bowl.
4. Add cinnamon and chopped mint and whisk in until spread evenly throughout the soup.
5. Cover and place in refrigerator for 1 to 2 hours.
6. Serve chilled.

YIELD: 4 servings (1 cup each)

NUTRITIONAL INFORMATION:
Calories 146.25
Protein .... 6.48 grams
Fat .... 0.4 grams
Carbs .... 29.1 grams

Vegetarian Chili

JACQUELYN WINDFELDT

INGREDIENTS:
1 medium-sized onion, minced
2 cloves garlic, minced
2 stalks celery, finely minced
1 bell pepper, chopped
1 teaspoon cumin
1 tablespoon chili powder
1 to 2 bay leaves
½ teaspoon oregano
½ teaspoon dried basil
2 cans (15 ounces each) of crushed tomatoes
¾ cup mushrooms, washed and chopped
1 zucchini, roughly chopped
¼ teaspoon cinnamon
1 can (15 ounces) black beans

METHOD:
1. Spray the bottom of a large pan with nonfat cooking spray and sauté onions, garlic, celery and bell peppers on medium-high until softened.
2. Add cumin, chili powder, bay leaves, oregano and basil and cook for 1 to 2 minutes longer.
3. Add tomatoes, mushrooms, zucchini and cinnamon.

4. Heat to boiling, then reduce heat to simmer and cook for 1 hour, covered.
5. Stir in beans and cook, uncovered, to desired thickness.
6. Season with salt and pepper to taste.

YIELD: 7 servings (1 cup each)

NUTRITIONAL INFORMATION:

Calories 75
Protein........... 3.28 grams
Fat .... 0.2 grams
Carbs .... 14.9 grams

SIDES AND SAUCES

Cranberry Sauce

DANIEL KIRSCHENBAUM

INGREDIENTS:

1 package (12 ounces) fresh cranberries
½ cup water
½ cup sugar substitute (check label of sugar substitute to make sure you use the equivalent of ½ cup of sugar)

METHOD:

1. Combine cranberries and water in a saucepan and heat until boiling. Boil for 15 minutes.
2. Remove pan from heat and let stand for 10 minutes.
3. Add sugar substitute to taste.

YIELD: 9 servings (¼ cup each)

NUTRITIONAL INFORMATION:

Calories 17
Protein........... 0 grams
Fat .... 0.01 grams
Carbs .... 4.24 grams

Very Low-Fat Mashed Potatoes
DAVID BURNS

INGREDIENTS:
2 pounds potatoes, peeled and quartered
½ cup fat-free sour cream
½ cup fat-free chicken broth
½ teaspoon salt
¼ teaspoon white pepper
½ teaspoon ground nutmeg (optional)

METHOD:
1. Put potatoes in a soup pot with ½ gallon of water and boil until tender.
2. Drain potatoes and transfer to a large mixing bowl.
3. Whip the potatoes on a low speed, and slowly add in the sour cream and chicken broth.
4. Add salt, pepper and nutmeg.
5. Increase speed of mixer and whip potatoes until desired consistency is reached.

YIELD:
8 servings (½ cup each)

NUTRITIONAL INFORMATION:
Calories 113
Protein........... 4.97 grams
Fat .... 0.17 grams
Carbs .... 22.87 grams

Simple Pasta Sauce
MEGAN O'REILLY

INGREDIENTS:
1 onion, chopped
1 teaspoon chopped garlic
½ teaspoon black pepper
1 teaspoon basil
1 teaspoon oregano
1 can (14.5 ounces) crushed tomatoes
½ teaspoon sweetener
1 can (14.5 ounces) diced tomatoes

METHOD:
1. Lightly spray pan with nonfat spray and sauté onion and garlic until onions are transparent.
2. Add spices while sautéing.
3. Add crushed tomatoes and sweetener and sauté a minute or so.

4. Add diced tomatoes, lower heat and simmer lightly for about an hour.

YIELD: 4 servings (½ cup each)

NUTRITIONAL INFORMATION:
Calories 63
Protein .... 1 gram
Fat .... 0 grams
Carbs .... 14.75 grams

Creamy Vegetable Pasta Sauce
JACQUELYN WINDFELDT

INGREDIENTS:
2 cups fat-free cottage cheese
5 tablespoons fat-free Parmesan cheese
¼ teaspoon red pepper flakes
2 tablespoons fat-free chicken or vegetable broth
1 medium-sized onion, chopped
½ teaspoon minced garlic
1 cup broccoli florets
1 cup cauliflower florets
1 small red bell pepper, sliced
1 large carrot, shredded
¼ pound sliced mushrooms

METHOD:
1. Combine cottage cheese, Parmesan cheese and red pepper flakes in a food processor or blender and mix until smooth and creamy.
2. In a skillet, mix together onion, garlic and broth and sauté at medium-high heat.
3. When onion and garlic are softened, add broccoli, cauliflower, red pepper and carrots and cook for about 6 minutes. Add mushrooms and cook until softened.
4. Stir in blended cheese mixture and cook on low heat for 10 minutes.

YIELD: 8 servings (½ cup each)

NUTRITIONAL INFORMATION:
Calories 64
Protein .... 9.5 grams
Fat .... 0 grams
Carbs .... 6.5 grams

Apple Oat Bread
MEGAN O'REILLY

INGREDIENTS:
1 cup white flour
1 cup wheat flour
1 teaspoon baking powder
¾ teaspoon salt
1 teaspoon baking soda
2 tablespoons brown sugar
2 cups oats
6 tablespoons maple syrup
1⅔ cup fat-free yogurt
1¼ cup hydrated apple

METHOD:
1. Preheat oven to 350 degrees.
2. Mix flours, baking powder, salt, baking soda, brown sugar and oats in a medium bowl.
3. In a separate bowl, mix together maple syrup, yogurt and hydrated apple.
4. Add the wet ingredients to the dry and combine until the dry are completely moistened. It should be a thick, sticky dough.
5. With minimal handling, scoop into bread pan and bake for 30 minutes.

YIELD: 6 servings (2 slices each)

NUTRITIONAL INFORMATION:
Calories 288
Protein .... 5.3 grams
Fat .... 1.4 grams
Carbs .... 63.2 grams

Cornbread
MEGAN O'REILLY

INGREDIENTS:
1 cup cornmeal
1 cup flour
½ teaspoon baking soda
½ teaspoon baking powder
½ teaspoon salt
1 cup fat-free buttermilk
½ cup egg whites

METHOD:
1. Preheat oven to 350 degrees.

2. Mix cornmeal, flour, baking soda, baking powder and salt in large bowl.
3. Combine buttermilk and egg whites in a second bowl.
4. Slowly add wet mixture to dry ingredients and combine until all of the flour mixture is moistened; pour into a lightly greased pan.
5. Bake for 30 minutes, or until cornbread is slightly browned (add chopped jalapeños or green chilies if desired).

YIELD: 8 slices

NUTRITIONAL INFORMATION:
Calories 131
Protein........... 4.4 grams
Fat .... 1 gram
Carbs............. 26.1 grams

Mango Marinade/Sauce
MEGAN O'REILLY

INGREDIENTS:
2 cups diced mango (fresh or frozen)
5 teaspoons fresh ginger, minced
5 tablespoons brown sugar
10 tablespoons cider vinegar (½ cup plus
        2 tablespoons)
1 teaspoon hot sauce
1 tablespoon fresh garlic

METHOD:
1. Purée all ingredients in a food processor.
2. Pour over fish, chicken or sliced tofu and bake.

YIELD: 8 servings (¼ cup each)

NUTRITIONAL INFORMATION:
Calories 64
Protein........... 0.4 grams
Fat .... 0 grams
Carbs............. 15.6 grams

Fat-Free Gravy
DAVID BURNS

INGREDIENTS:
2 cups fat-free chicken broth
2 tablespoons cornstarch
½ teaspoon sage
Dash Kitchen Bouquet

METHOD:
1. Heat to boil chicken broth.
2. While the broth is heating, in a small mixing bowl combine cornstarch with enough very cold water (about 1 tablespoon) to moisten all of it.
3. Slowly pour cornstarch mixture into the chicken broth and mix until desired thickness is reached. Note: the gravy will appear rather translucent.
4. Add sage and a dash of Kitchen Bouquet for color.

YIELD: 10 servings (1½ ounces each)

NUTRITIONAL INFORMATION:
Calories......... 5
Protein........... 0 grams
Fat.................. 0 grams
Carbs............. 1.25 grams

Orange Cranberry Sauce
DANIEL KIRSCHENBAUM

INGREDIENTS:
¾ cup sugar substitute (check label of sugar substitute to make sure you use the equivalent of ¾ cup sugar)
1 cup water
3 cups fresh or frozen cranberries (a 12-ounce bag)
1 large orange, peeled and cubed (1-inch squares)

METHOD:
1. In a saucepan, mix sugar substitute and water until sugar substitute is dissolved.
2. Bring the sugar water to a boil, then add the cranberries, return to a boil and reduce heat.
3. Add the oranges to the pan and boil gently, stirring occasionally, for 10 minutes.
4. Cool to room temperature and then refrigerate.

YIELD: 9 servings (¼ cup each)

NUTRITIONAL INFORMATION:
Calories......... 31
Fat.................. 0 grams
Protein........... 0 grams
Carbs............. 7.75 grams

Baba Ganouj (Eggplant Dip)

JACQUELYN WINDFELDT

INGREDIENTS:

2 medium-sized eggplants
2 to 3 lemons, juiced
¾ cup Tahini*
6 tablespoons minced garlic
½ cup chopped parsley
2 teaspoons salt
½ cup chopped scallions (optional)
Black pepper to taste
1 cup fat-free plain yogurt

METHOD:

1. Preheat oven to 400 degrees.
2. Cut off the stems of both eggplants and prick each eggplant several times with a fork.
3. Place the eggplants directly onto the oven rack and cook for approximately 45 minutes, or until the skin is shriveled and the eggplant is soft.
4. Remove eggplants from the oven and set aside until they are cool enough to handle.
5. Once they have cooled, cut along the length of your eggplants and scoop their cooked insides out.
6. Discard skins and put eggplant into a food processor or blender with remaining ingredients.
7. Blend until smooth and creamy. Serve as a dip with fat-free crackers, mini pita bread or raw vegetables.

YIELD: 24 servings (2 ounces/2 teaspoons each)

NUTRITIONAL INFORMATION:

Calories 35
Protein .... 1.2 grams
Fat .... 1.8 grams
Carbs .... 3.5 grams

*NOTE: Tahini is a paste made of crushed sesame seeds. It can be purchased at a Middle Eastern grocery store or in the international foods section of your local grocery store.

Hummus (Chickpea Dip)

JACQUELYN WINDFELDT

INGREDIENTS:

1 can (16 ounces) chickpeas (garbanzo beans)
4 cloves minced garlic (more if a stronger taste is desired)
2 tablespoons Tahini
2 tablespoons lemon juice
⅓ teaspoon cumin
⅓ teaspoon black pepper
Dash red pepper
⅔ teaspoon of salt (to taste)

METHOD:

1. Combine all of the ingredients in a food processor or blender and mix until smooth. It may be necessary to add moisture to the mixture; warm water, fat-free milk or fat-free yogurt are acceptable options.
2. Additional ingredients, such as roasted red peppers, sun-dried tomatoes, or herbs may be added for a different twist. This recipe can also be prepared with black beans. Nutritional information will be different.
3. Serve with fresh vegetables or pita bread.

YIELD:

8 servings (2 ounces /2 teaspoons each)

NUTRITIONAL INFORMATION:

Calories 47
Protein........... 4 grams
Fat .... 1.7 grams
Carbs .... 3.95 grams

Fat-Free Garlic Bread

DANIEL KIRSCHENBAUM

INGREDIENTS:

1 loaf French bread
30 to 40 squirts of fat-free butter spray
2 teaspoons garlic salt

METHOD:

1. Preheat oven to 400 degrees.
2. Slice the bread lengthwise and open up so that the crust side is facing down.
3. Spray the upturned side liberally with the fat-free butter spray.
4. Sprinkle the garlic salt to coat one side lightly.

5. Place on a cookie sheet and cook at 400 degrees for 15 minutes, until underside is crispy.

YIELD: 5 servings (2 ounces each)

NUTRITIONAL INFORMATION:
Calories 130
Protein .... 4 grams
Fat .... 0 grams
Carbs .... 27 grams

Sweetpotatoes*

DANIEL KIRSCHENBAUM

HOW TO CHOOSE: Select firm, well-rounded sweetpotatoes with clean, smooth skin. Watch out for soft spots, obvious bruises and signs of decay.

HOW TO USE: Do not refrigerate sweetpotatoes unless they are cooked. Cold temperatures can cause them to become bitter. Instead, store sweetpotatoes in a cool (55°F is ideal), dry place. I use newly purchased sweetpotatoes within a week or two if possible. The North Carolina Sweetpotato Commission recommends using only a stainless steel knife to cut sweetpotatoes. They also advise placing them in cold water while preparing them to prevent darkening.

BASIC COOKING ADVICE:
- To bake: Prick the skin with a fork and bake at 400 degrees for forty to fifty minutes or until soft to the touch.
- To microwave: Prick the skin several times and microwave on high power for six to eight minutes for an 8-ounce sweetpotato.
- To boil: Place whole sweetpotatoes in boiling water and cook for about forty minutes.
- To steam: Bring 1½ inches of water to a boil in a steamer. Place whole, unpeeled sweetpotatoes in a steam basket and cook until tender (forty to fifty minutes for an 8-ounce sweetpotato). When peeled and cut into 1-inch cubes as an alternative, they will cook in thirty minutes.

- Uncooked: Peel and cut into sticks and dip into your favorite dip.

TYPICAL TOPPINGS:

Many great toppings can enhance the flavor and variety of sweetpotatoes. Consider trying the following:

- Salsa, particularly fruit salsas
- Cinnamon-flavored applesauce
- Vanilla-flavored fat-free yogurt with cinnamon
- Fat-free imitation butter spread and cinnamon sugar (cinnamon + sweetener)
- Sweet and sour sauce
- Mandarin oranges with crushed pineapple
- Honey mustard combinations (including honey + Dijon mustard)
- Barbecue sauce
- Veggie chili

NUTRITIONAL INFORMATION:

1 sweetpotato (5 inches by 2 inches), baked in skin
Calories 118
Protein........... 1 grams
Fat .... 0.1 gram
Carbs .... 27.7 grams

* Adapted from materials provided by the North Carolina Sweetpotato Commission; used with permission.

Apple-Baked Sweetpotatoes*

INGREDIENTS:

6 medium-sized sweetpotatoes
⅓ cup brown sugar
1 tablespoon flour
1 teaspoon salt
2 tablespoons orange juice
3 apples, peeled and sliced

METHOD:

1. Preheat oven to 350 degrees.
2. Bake sweetpotatoes until soft, peel, cut lengthwise and slice.
3. In a small bowl, combine sugar, flour, salt and orange juice.
4. Layer ingredients in casserole: first layer

sweetpotatoes, second layer apples, third
layer sugar mixture.
5. Bake for 1 hour.

YIELD: 6 servings

NUTRITIONAL INFORMATION:
Calories 219
Protein .... 2.3 grams
Fat .... 0.1 grams
Carbs .... 52.5 grams

* Isabel Raci's assistance in developing and testing some of the sweetpotato recipes is acknowledged gratefully.

Curried Sweetpotato Salad with Fruit Medley

INGREDIENTS:
2 pounds sweetpotatoes, peeled and diced
1 cup fat-free yogurt
1 tablespoon curry powder
1 piece (1 inch) fresh ginger root, minced
1 teaspoon brown sugar
¼ cup golden raisins
⅛ cup dried cherries
⅛ cup black raisins
4 green onions, chopped
Salt to taste
Freshly ground pepper to taste

METHOD:
1. Place potatoes in large pot. Cover with cold
water and bring to a boil. Reduce heat and
simmer potatoes for about 7 minutes or
until tender. Drain and set aside.
2. Combine yogurt, curry powder, ginger root
and brown sugar in medium bowl; add potatoes, fruit, onions and salt and pepper to
taste; toss to coat.

YIELD: 6 servings (8 ounces each)

NUTRITIONAL INFORMATION:
Calories 150
Protein .... 5 grams
Fat .... 0.1 grams
Carbs .... 32.5 grams

Orange-Lime Sweetpotatoes

INGREDIENTS:
1 cup chopped onion
1 teaspoon garlic
1 pound sweetpotato pieces (1-inch squares)
1 cup orange juice
¼ cup lime juice
Salt and pepper to taste

METHOD:
1. Spray a skillet with nonfat cooking spray and sauté onion and garlic.
2. Add sweetpotato and juices to skillet.
3. Bring to a boil, reduce heat and simmer until sauce thickens.
4. Add salt, pepper to taste.

YIELD:
6 servings (4 ounces each)

NUTRITIONAL INFORMATION:
Calories 67
Protein .... 1 gram
Fat .... 0.1 grams
Carbs .... 15.75 grams

Siam Sweetpotatoes

INGREDIENTS:
1½ pounds sweetpotatoes, peeled and cut into ½-inch pieces
Nonfat cooking spray
1 onion, chopped
2 cloves garlic, minced
1½ teaspoons grated fresh ginger root
½ teaspoon Thai curry powder
¼ teaspoon red pepper flakes
1 can (12 ounces) evaporated skim milk
¼ teaspoon coconut extract
½ cup water
½ teaspoon (or less) salt
1 cup frozen green peas, thawed
1 tablespoon grated lemon peel
4 cups hot cooked white rice
¼ cup chopped fresh cilantro
2 tablespoons "Better 'N Peanut Butter" or "Peanut Wonder" (soy-based low-fat substitutes for peanut butter)

METHOD:

1. In a large saucepan, cover the sweetpotatoes with water and heat until boiling. Cook 10 minutes, drain and set aside.
2. Spray the bottom of a large skillet with non-fat cooking spray; add the onion and sauté until tender.
3. Add the garlic, ginger, curry powder and pepper flakes; cook, stirring occasionally, 3 minutes.
4. Add the cooked sweetpotatoes, evaporated milk, coconut extract, water and salt; heat to boiling.
5. Reduce the heat, cover and simmer for 20 minutes or until the potatoes are tender.
6. Remove from heat and stir in the peas and lemon peel.
7. Place the hot cooked rice in a serving dish and top with the potato mixture; add peanut butter substitute; sprinkle with cilantro and serve.

YIELD: 6 servings (8 ounces each)

NUTRITIONAL INFORMATION: Calories 289
                          Protein .... 9.67 grams
                          Fat .... 0.1 grams
                          Carbs .... 62.6 grams

Sweetpotato Cakes

INGREDIENTS:

2 carrots, shredded
1 medium-sized sweetpotato, shredded
½ cup chopped onions
2 cloves garlic, minced
⅓ cup black bean dry dip mix
½ cup bread crumbs
⅛ teaspoon ground fennel
½ teaspoon cumin
½ teaspoon coriander
¼ teaspoon Spike Seasoning
¼ cup egg substitute
⅛ teaspoon cayenne
½ to ⅓ cup rolled oats
¼ teaspoon sesame seeds

½ cup frozen peas
1 heaped tablespoon shredded fat-free mozzarella
1 tablespoon dried parsley

METHOD:

1. In a large bowl, mix all ingredients together vigorously. Form into small cakes about 3 to 3½ inches in diameter.
2. Spray a nonstick frying pan with nonfat spray cooking oil.
3. Cook cakes on medium heat for about 10 to 15 minutes, turning every few minutes; they should be lightly browned and cooked through.
4. Serve with a dollop of fat-free sour cream and garnish with a bit of parsley.

YIELD:

4 servings (6 ounces each)

NUTRITIONAL INFORMATION:

Calories 90
Protein........... 5 grams
Fat .... 0.1 grams
Carbs .... 17.5 grams

Sweetpotato Carrot Salad

INGREDIENTS:

1 teaspoon fresh lemon juice
2 teaspoons fat-free mayonnaise
1 cup chopped fresh pineapple
Pinch of salt
1 cup raisins
2 teaspoons grated fresh ginger
2 large carrots, shredded
1 medium-sized sweetpotato, shredded

METHOD:

1. Purée the lemon juice with the mayonnaise and a few chunks of the pineapple and salt. Set aside.
2. Mix together the raisins, ginger, remaining pineapple, shredded carrots and sweetpotato.
3. Pour the mayonnaise mixture over this, toss and let marinate for half an hour.
4. Chill.

YIELD:

4 servings (6 ounces each)

NUTRITIONAL INFORMATION:
Calories 186
Protein .... 2.2 grams
Fat .... 0.1 grams
Carbs .... 44.3 grams

Sweetpotato Pancakes

INGREDIENTS:
4 cups (packed) coarsely grated sweetpotatoes
    (approximately 1 large or 2 medium-sized)
½ cup grated onion
3 to 4 tablespoons lemon juice
1 teaspoon salt
Black pepper to taste
6 whipped egg whites
⅓ cup flour
¼ cup minced parsley (optional)

METHOD:
1. Combine all ingredients and mix well.
2. Spray a nonstick frying pan with nonfat cooking spray and heat.
3. Use a non-slotted spoon to transfer the batter to the pan, patting the batter down into thin pancakes. Brown on both sides and serve hot with toppings (fat-free sour cream or yogurt; applesauce).

YIELD:
4 pancakes

NUTRITIONAL INFORMATION:
Calories 135
Protein .... 3 grams
Fat .... 0.1 grams
Carbs .... 30.75 grams

Sweetpotato Pie

INGREDIENTS:
4 egg whites, beaten
¾ cup sugar
2 cups mashed sweetpotatoes
¾ cup evaporated skim milk
1 teaspoon vanilla extract
¼ teaspoon salt
½ teaspoon cinnamon
½ teaspoon nutmeg

METHOD:

1. Preheat oven to 375 degrees.
2. In a large bowl, mix together egg whites and sugar; add sweetpotatoes and mix well.
3. Stir in milk, vanilla, salt, cinnamon and nutmeg, making sure all ingredients are thoroughly mixed.
4. Pour into a greased (nonfat) glass pie plate.
5. Bake for 40 minutes or until knife inserted comes out clean.

YIELD:

8 servings (4 ounces each)

NUTRITIONAL INFORMATION:

Calories 143
Protein .... 2.75 grams
Fat .... 0.1 grams
Carbs .... 33 grams

Sweetpotato Pudding

INGREDIENTS:

2 cups mashed cooked sweetpotato
½ cup firmly packed brown sugar
4 egg whites
¾ cup unsweetened orange juice
¼ teaspoon ground nutmeg
¼ teaspoon ground cloves
Dash of salt
2 tablespoons sugar
Nonfat cooking spray

METHOD:

1. Preheat oven to 350 degrees.
2. Beat egg whites (at room temperature) until foamy; add salt and beat until soft peaks form; add sugar; beat until stiff peaks form.
3. Combine potato, brown sugar and egg whites in a large bowl; stir well.
4. Gradually add orange juice, nutmeg and cloves; stir well and set aside.
5. Fold egg whites into potato mixture.
6. Pour mixture into a ½-quart baking dish coated with cooking spray; place baking dish in a large, shallow pan.
7. Pour hot water in outer pan to a depth of 1 inch.
8. Bake for 1 hour or until center is set and edges are browned.

9. Remove dish from water; let cool 15 minutes
before serving.

YIELD: 10 servings (4 ounces each)

NUTRITIONAL INFORMATION:
Calories 100
Protein .... 2.5 grams
Fat .... 0.1 grams
Carbs .... 22.5 grams

DESSERTS

Pumpkin Pudding Pie
DANIEL KIRSCHENBAUM

INGREDIENTS:
1 can (30 ounces) Libby's Easy Pumpkin Pie Mix
½ cup Egg Beaters or egg whites
1 cup evaporated skim milk
2 pie shells in aluminum pans (9-inch)

METHOD:
1. Preheat oven to 425 degrees.
2. Mix pumpkin pie mix, egg substitute and
evaporated milk in large bowl.
3. Pour into pie shells.
4. Bake in oven for 15 minutes.
5. Reduce temperature to 350 degrees and
bake another 50 to 60 minutes or until knife
inserted in center comes out clean.
6. Cool for 2 hours or refrigerate.
7. Serve plain or with fat-free Cool Whip (adds
15 calories per 2 tablespoons to nutritional
information below).

YIELD: 12 servings (3½ ounces each)

NUTRITIONAL INFORMATION:
Calories 97
Protein .... 3.2 grams
Fat .... 0.4 grams
Carbs .... 20 grams

Oatmeal Cookies

JACQUELYN WINDFELDT

INGREDIENTS:

¾ cup silken tofu
1½ cups brown sugar
¼ cup apple butter
¼ cup egg substitute
1 teaspoon vanilla
1½ cups flour
1 teaspoon baking soda
1 teaspoon cinnamon
½ teaspoon salt
3 cups oats
1 cup raisins

METHOD:

1. Preheat oven to 350 degrees.
2. Combine silken tofu, brown sugar, apple butter, egg substitute and vanilla in a food processor and mix until well blended.
3. In a separate bowl, mix flour, baking soda, cinnamon and salt and stir until evenly blended.
4. Slowly stir the tofu mixture into the dry ingredients.
5. When dry mix is moistened, add oats and raisins and continue to stir until oats and raisins are blended into mix.
6. Spray cookie sheets with nonfat cooking spray and place tablespoon-sized balls of dough onto sheet.
7. Flatten with a spoon and bake for 30 to 35 minutes or until they begin to brown.

YIELD:

24 cookies (2 cookies per serving)

NUTRITIONAL INFORMATION:
(PER SERVING)

Calories 97
Protein .... 3 grams
Fat .... 1.8 grams
Carbs .... 17 grams

REFERENCES

CHAPTER 1: THE WELLSPRING PLAN: 8 STEPS TO SUCCESS

Baker, R. C., & Kirschenbaum, D. S. (1998). Weight control during the holidays: Highly consistent self-monitoring as a potentially useful coping mechanism. *Health Psychology, 17*, 367–370.

Baumeister, R. F., Heatherton, T. F., & Tice, D. M. (1994). *Losing Control: How and Why People Fail at Self-Regulation*. San Diego, CA: Academic Press.

Boutelle, K. N., & Kirschenbaum, D. S. (1998). Further support for consistent self-monitoring as a vital component of successful weight control. *Obesity Research, 6*, 219–224.

Ericsson, K. A., & Charness, N. (1994). Expert performance: Its structure and acquisition. *American Psychologist, 49*, 725–747.

Kirschenbaum, D. S. (1987). Self-regulatory failure: A review with clinical implications. *Clinical Psychology Review, 7*, 77–104.

Kirschenbaum, D. S. (1994). *Weight loss through persistence: Making science work for you*. Oakland, CA: New Harbinger.

Kirschenbaum, D. S. (2000). *The 9 Truths about Weight Loss*. New York: Holt.

Kirschenbaum, D. S., & Karoly, P. (1977). When self-regulation fails: Tests of some preliminary hypotheses. *Journal of Consulting and Clinical Psychology, 45,* 1116–1125.

McGuire, M. T., Wing, R. R., Klem, M. L., Lang, W. & Hill, J. O. (1999). What predicts weight regain in a group of successful weight losers? *Journal of Consulting and Clinical Psychology, 67,* 177–185.

McGuire, M. T., Wing, R. R., Klem, M. L., & Hill, J. O. (1999). Behavioral strategies of individuals who have maintained long-term weight losses. *Obesity Research, 7,* 334–341.

Perri, M. G., Anton, S. D. et al. (2002). Adherence to exercise prescriptions: Effects of prescribing moderate versus higher levels of intensity and frequency. *Health Psychology, 21,* 452–458.

Perri, M. G., Nezu, A. M., & Viegener, B. J. (1992). *Improving the Long-Term Management of Obesity: Theory, Research, and Clinical Guidelines.* New York: John Wiley.

Sperduto, W. A., Thompson, H. S., & O'Brien, R. M. (1986). The effect of target behavior monitoring on weight loss and completion rate in a behavior modification program for weight reduction. *Addictive Behaviors, 11,* 337–340.

Stice, E. (1998). Prospective relation of dieting behaviors to weight change in a community sample of adolescents. *Behavior Therapy, 29,* 277–297.

Wing, R. R., & Hill, J. O. (2001). Successful weight loss maintenance. *Annual Review of Nutrition, 21,* 323–341.

CHAPTER 2: STEP 1: MAKE THE DECISION

Hubbel, M. A., Duncan, B. L., & Miller, S. D. (1999). (Eds.). *The heart & soul of change: What works in therapy.* Washington, D.C.: American Psychological Association.

Ikemi, Y., & Nakagawa, S. (1962). A psychosomatic study of contagious dermatitis. *Kyosu Journal of Medical Science, 13,* 335–350.

Janis, I. L., & Mann, L. (1977). *Decision making: A psychological analysis of conflict, choice and commitment.* New York: The Free Press.

Kirsch, I. (1990). Changing expectations. *A key to effective psychotherapy.* Pacific Grove, CA: Brooks/Cole.

Kirschenbaum, D. S., Fitzgibbon, M. L., Martino, S., Conviser, J. H., Rosendahl, E. H., & Laatsch, L. (1992). Stages of change in successful weight control: A clinically derived model. *Behavior Therapy, 23,* 623–635.

Meichenbaum, D., & Turk, D. C. (1987). *Facilitating Treatment Adherence: A practitioner's guidebook.* New York: Plenum.

Nelson, L. R., & Furst, M. L. (1972). An objective study of the effects of expectation on competitive performance. *Journal of Psychology, 81,* 69–72.

Shapiro, A. K. (1978). Placebo effects in medicine, psychotherapy and psychoanalysis. In A. P. Bergin & S. L. Garfield (Eds.). *Handbook of Psychotherapy and Behavior Change: An empirical analysis.* New York: John Wiley.

Vincent, P. (1971). Factors influencing patient noncompliance: A theoretical approach. *Nursing Research, 20,* 509–516.

CHAPTER 3: STEP 2: KNOW THE ENEMY—YOUR BIOLOGY

Barnard, N. D., Akhtar, A., & Nicholson, A. (1995). Factors that facilitate compliance to lower fat intake. *Archives of Family Medicine, 4,* 153–158.

Bessesen, D. H., Rupp, C. L., & Eckel, R. H. (1995). Dietary fat is shunted away from oxidation, toward storage in obese Zucker rats. *Obesity Research, 3,* 179–189.

Blass, E. (1989). Opioids, sweets and a mechanism for positive affect: Broad motivational implications. In J. Dobbing (Ed.) *Sweetness.* New York: Springer-Verlag.

Blundell, J. E., Burley, V. J., Cotton, J. R., & Lawton, C. L. (1993). Dietary fat in the control of energy intake: Evaluating the effects of fat on meal size and postmeal satiety. *American Journal of Clinical Nutrition, 57,* 772S–778S.

Boozer, C. N., Brasseur, A., & Atkinson, R. L. (1993). Dietary fat affects weight loss and adiposity during energy restriction in rats. *American Journal of Clinical Nutrition, 58,* 846–852.

Dobbing, J. (Ed.). (1987). *Sweetness.* New York: Springer-Verlag.

Epstein, L. H., Valoski, A., Wing, R. R., & McCurley, J. (1994). Ten-year outcomes of behavioral family-based treatment for childhood obesity. *Health Psychology, 13,* 373–383.

Geiselman, P. J., & Novin, D. (1982). The role of carbohydrates in appetite, hunger and obesity. *Appetite, 3,* 203–223.

Hartigan, K. J., Baker-Strauch, D., & Morris, G. W. (1982). Perceptions of the causes of obesity and responsiveness to treatment. *Journal of Counseling Psychology, 29,* 478–485.

Hill, J. O., Drougas, H., & Peters, J. C. (1993). Obesity treatment: Can diet composition play a role? *Annals of Internal Medicine, 119,* 694–697.

Jeffery, R. W., Hellerstedt, W. L., French, S. A. & Baxter, J. E. (1995). A randomized trial of counseling for fat restriction versus calorie restriction in the treatment of obesity. *International Journal of Obesity, 19,* 132–137.

Jeffery, R. W., Wing, R. R., & Mayer, R. R. (1998). Are smaller weight losses or more achievable weight loss goals better in the long term for obese patients? *Journal of Consulting and Clinical Psychology, 66,* 641–645.

Kirschenbaum, D. S., et al. (1992). Stages of change in successful weight control: A clinically derived model. *Behavior Therapy, 23*, 623–635.

Kramer, F. M., Jeffery, R. W., Forster, J. L., & Snell, M. K. (1989). Long-term follow-up of behavioral treatment for obesity: Patterns of weight regain among men and women. *International Journal of Obesity, 13*, 123–136.

Liebman, B. (2004). Fat: More than just a lump of lard. *Nutrition Action Health Letter, 31*, 1–6.

Ravussin, E., & Swinburn, B. A. (1993). Energy metabolism. In A. J. Stunkard & T. A. Wadden (Eds.) *Obesity: Theory & Therapy, Second Edition*. New York: Raven Press.

Sims, E. Z. H., Danforth, E., et al. (1973). Endocrine and metabolic effects of experimental obesity in man. *Recent Progress in Hormone Research, 29*, 457–487.

Staff Writer (1996). Weight loss news that's easy to stomach. *Tufts University Diet & Nutrition Letter, 14*.

Stunkard, A. J. (1958). The management of obesity. *New York State Journal of Medicine, 58*, 79–87.

Wadden, T. A. (1993). Treatment of obesity by moderate and severe caloric restriction: Results of clinical research trials. *Annals of Internal Medicine, 119*, 688–693.

Wadden, T. A. et al. (1997). Lifestyle modification in the pharmacologic treatment of obesity: A pilot investigation of a potential primary care approach. *Obesity Research, 5*, 218–226.

CHAPTER 4: STEP 3: EAT TO LOSE

Barnard, N. D., Akhtar, A., & Nicholson, A. (1995). Factors that facilitate compliance to lower fat intake. *Archives of Family Medicine, 4*, 153–158.

Bessesen, D. H., Rupp, C. L., & Eckel, R. H. (1995). Dietary fat is shunted away from oxidation, toward storage in obese Zucker rats. *Obesity Research, 3*, 179–189.

Boozer, C. N., Brasseur, A., & Atkinson, R. L. (1993). Dietary fat affects weight loss and adiposity during energy restriction in rats. *American Journal of Clinical Nutrition, 58*, 846–852.

Campbell, T. C. with Campbell, T. M. (2005). *The China Study: Startling implications for diet, weight loss and long-term health*. Dallas, TX: BenBella Books.

Dobbing, J. (Ed.). (1987). *Sweetness*. NY: Springer-Verlag.

Geiselman, P. J., & Novin, D. (1982). The role of carbohydrates in appetite, hunger and obesity. *Appetite, 3*, 203–223.

Harris, J. K., French, S. A., Jeffery, R. W., McGovern, P., & Wing, R. R. (1994). Dietary and physical activity correlates of long-term weight loss. *Obesity Research, 2*, 307–313.

Hill, J. O., Drougas, H., & Peters, J. C. (1993). Obesity treatment: Can diet composition play a role? *Annals of Internal Medicine, 119*, 694–697.

Jeffery, R. W., Hellerstedt, W. L., French, S. A. & Baxter, J. E. (1995). A randomized trial of counseling for fat restriction versus calorie restriction in the treatment of obesity. *International Journal of Obesity, 19*, 132–137.

Staff writers (December, 1998). *Diet and cancer: The Big Picture, 25*, 10.

Staff writers (December, 1998). Seven excuses for not eating better (that don't hold up under close scrutiny). *Tufts University Health & Nutritional Letter.*

Stice, E. (1998). Prospective relation of dieting behaviors to weight change in a community sample of adolescents. *Behavior Therapy, 29*, 277–297.

Thayer, R. E. (1987). Energy, tiredness and tension effects of a sugar snack versus moderate exercise. *Journal of Personality and Social Psychology, 52*, 119–125.

CHAPTER 6: STEP 5: MOVE TO LOSE

Baechle, T. R., & Groves, B. R. (1992). *Weight Training: Steps to Success.* Champaign, IL: Leisure Press.

Blair, S. N. (1991). *Living with exercise.* Dallas, TX: American Health Publishing Co.

Blair, S. N. (1991). Weight loss through physical activity. *Weight Control Digest, 1*, 17, 20–24.

Carpenter, R. A. (2004). Getting in step with counters. *Weight Management Newsletter of the American Dietetic Association, 1*, 1–2.

Curless, M. R. (1992). Only the fit stay young. *Self*, September, 180–181.

Dishman, R. K. (Ed.). (1988). *Exercise adherence: Its impact on public health.* Champaign, IL: Human Kinetics Publishers.

Donahoe, C. P., Jr., Lin, D. H., Kirschenbaum, D. S., & Keesey, R. E. (1984). Metabolic consequences of dieting and exercise in the treatment of obesity. *Journal of Consulting and Clinical Psychology, 52*, 827–836.

Gavin, J. (1991). *The Exercise Habit: Your personal road map to developing a lifelong exercise commitment.* Champaign, IL: Human Kinetics Publishers.

Hall, C., Figueroa, A., Fernhall, B., & Kanaley, J. A. (2004). Energy expenditure of walking and running: Comparison with prediction equations. *Medicine & Science in Sports & Exercise, 36*, 2128–2134.

Heil, J. (1993). *Psychology of Sport Injury.* Champaign, IL: Human Kinetics Publishers.

Kendzierski, D. and Johnson, W. (1993). Excuses, excuses, excuses: A cognitive behavioral approach to exercise implementation. *Journal of Sport and Exercise Psychology, 15*, 207–219.

Kirschenbaum, D. S. (1998). *Mind Matters: Seven Steps to Smarter Sport Performance*. Carmel, IN: Cooper Publishing Group.

Kusinitz, I., Fin, M. and Editors of *Consumer Reports* Books. (1983). *Physical Fitness for Practically Everybody: The Consumer's Union Report on exercise*. Mount Vernon, NY: Consumers Union.

Latella, F. S., Conkling, W. and Editors of *Consumers Reports* Books. (1989). *Get in Shape, Stay in Shape*. New York: Consumer Reports Books.

Rippe, J. M. and Amend, P. (1992). *The exercise exchange program*. New York: Simon & Schuster.

Vickery, S. & Moffat, M. (1999). *The American Physical Therapy Association Book of Body Maintenance and Repair*. New York: Owl Books.

Chapter 7: Step 6: Self-Monitor and Plan Consistently

Baker, R. C., & Kirschenbaum, D. S. (1993). Self-monitoring may be necessary for successful weight control. *Behavior Therapy, 24*, 377–394.

Baker, R. C., & Kirschenbaum, D. S. (1998). Weight control during the holidays: Highly consistent self-monitoring as a potentially useful coping mechanism. *Health Psychology, 17*, 367–370.

Baumeister, R. F., Heatherton, T. F., & Tice, D. M. (1994). *Losing Control: How and Why People Fail at Self-Regulation*. San Diego, CA: Academic Press.

Boutelle, K. N., & Kirschenbaum, D. S. (1998). Further support for consistent self-monitoring as a vital component of successful weight control. *Obesity Research, 6*, 219–224.

Boutelle, K. N., Kirschenbaum, D. S., Baker, R. C., & Mitchell, M. E. (1999). How can obese weight controllers minimize weight gain during the high risk holiday season? By self-monitoring very consistently. *Health Psychology, 18*, 364–368.

Carver, C. S., & Scheier, M. F. (1990). Origins and functions of positive and negative affect: A control-process view. *Psychological Review, 97*, 19–35.

Kanfer, F. H., & Karoly, P. (1972). Self-control: A behavioristic excursion into the lion's den. *Behavior Therapy, 3*, 398–416.

Kirschenbaum, D. S. (1987). Self-regulatory failure: A review with clinical implications. *Clinical Psychology Review, 7*, 77–104.

Perri, M. G., Nezu, A. M., & Viegener, B. J. (1992). *Improving the Long-Term Management of Obesity: Theory, Research and Clinical Guidelines*. New York: John Wiley & Sons.

Schlundt, D. G., Sbrocco, T., & Bell, C. (1989). Identification of high-risk situations in a behavioral weight loss program: Application of the relapse prevention model. *International Journal of Obesity, 13*, 223–234.

Sperduto, W. A., Thompson, H. S., & O'Brien, R. M. (1986). The effect of target behavior monitoring on weight loss and completion rate in a behavior modification program for weight reduction. *Addictive Behaviors, 11,* 337–340.

Weinberg, R. S. (1988). *The Mental Advantage: Developing Your Psychological Skills in Tennis.* Champaign, IL: Leisure Press.

CHAPTER 8: STEP 7: UNDERSTAND AND MANAGE STRESS—WITH AND WITHOUT FOOD

Alberti, R. E. and Emmons, M. L. (1990). *Your Perfect Right: A Guide to Assertive Living* (6th ed.). San Luis Obispo, CA: Impact Publishers.

American Psychiatric Association. (1987). *Diagnostic and statistical manual of mental disorders* (3rd ed. rev.). Washington, D.C.

Barlow, D. H. and Rapee, R. M. (1991). *Mastering Stress: A Lifestyle Approach.* Dallas, TX: American Health Publishing Company.

Beckfield, D. F. (1994). *Master Your Panic and Take Back Your Life!* San Luis Obispo, CA: Impact Publishers.

Bernstein, D. A. and Borkovec, D. T. (1973). *Progressive Relaxation Training: A Manual for the Helping Professions.* Champaign, IL: Research Press.

Birkedahl, N. (1991). *Older & Wiser: A Workbook for Coping With Aging.* Oakland, CA: New Harbinger Publications, Inc.

Bourne, E. J. (1990). *The Anxiety & Phobia Workbook.* Oakland, CA: New Harbinger Publications, Inc.

Burns, D. E. (1989). *The Feeling Good Handbook: Using the new mood therapy in everyday life.* New York: William Morrow & Company.

Cautela, J. R. and Groden, J. (1991). *Relaxation: A Comprehensive Manual for Adults, Children, and Children With Special Needs.* Champaign, IL: Research Press.

Davis, M., Eshelman, E. R. and McKay, M. (1995). *The Relaxation & Stress Reduction Workbook* (4th ed.). Oakland, CA: New Harbinger Publications, Inc.

Ellis, A. and Harper, R. A. (1975). *New Guide to Rational Living.* Hollywood, CA: Wilshire Book Co.

Grasha, A. F. and Kirschenbaum, D. S. (1986). *Adjustment and Competence: Concepts and Applications.* Minneapolis, MN: West Publishing Company.

Harp, D., with Feldman, N. (1990). *The new three minute mediator.* Oakland, CA: New Harbinger Publications, Inc.

Holmes, T. H. and Rahe, R. H. (1967). The social readjustment rating scale. *Journal of Psychosomatic Research, 11,* 216.

Jacobson, E. (1929). *Progressive relaxation.* Chicago: University of Chicago Press.

Kirschenbaum, D. S. (1998). Using sport psychology to improve health psychology outcomes. *The Health Psychologist, 20,* 16–17, 22–23.

Kirschenbaum, D. S., & Wittrock, D. A. (1990). Still searching for effective criticism inoculation procedures. *Journal of Applied Sport Psychology, 2,* 175–185.

Klarreich, S. H. (1990). *Work with stress: A practical guide to emotional well-being on the job.* New York: Brunner/Mazel.

Marks, I. M. (1978). *Living With Fear: Understanding and Coping With Anxiety.* New York: McGraw-Hill.

McKay, M. and Fanning, P. (1993). *Time Out from Stress* (two ten-minute cassettes). Oakland, CA: New Harbinger Publications, Inc.

Meichenbaum, D. (1985). *Stress Inoculation Training.* New York: Pergamon.

Paine, W. S. (Ed.). (1982). Job Stress and Burnout. Beverly Hills, CA: Sage Publications.

Stevens, J. O. (1971). *Awareness: Exploring, Experimenting, Experiencing.* Moab, UT: Real People Press.

Tubesing, N. L. and Tubesing, D. H. (1990). *Structured Exercises in Stress Management.* Vols. 1–4, Duluth, MN: Whole Person Press.

Zilberg, N. J., Weiss, D. S. and Horowitz, M. J. (1982). Impact of Event Scale: A Cross-Validation Study. *Journal of Consulting and Clinical Psychology, 50,* 407–414.

CHAPTER 9: STEP 8: USE SLUMP BUSTERS TO OVERCOME SLUMPS

Bray, G. A. (1995). Pharmacologic treatment of obesity. *Obesity Research, 3,* Supplement 4.

Greenway, G. (1992). Non-prescription medications for weight control: A review. *American Journal of Clinical Nutrition, 55,* 203–205.

Kirschenbaum, D. S. (1988). Treating adult obesity in 1988: Evolution of a modern program. *The Behavior Therapist, 11,* 3–6.

Kirschenbaum, D. S. (1992). Elements of effective weight control programs: Implications for exercise and sport psychology. *Journal of Applied Sport Psychology, 4,* 77–93.

Kirschenbaum, D. S. and Tomarken, A. J. (1982). On facing the generalization problem: The study of self-regulatory failure. In P. C. Kendall (Ed.) *Advances in cognitive-behavioral research and therapy,* Vol. 1. New York: Academic Press.

Marlatt, G. A. and Gordon, J. R. (Eds.). (1985). *Relapse Prevention: Maintenance Strategies in the Treatment of Addictive Behaviors.* New York: Guilford Press.

National Institutes of Health. (1992). *Methods for voluntary weight loss and control: Technology Assessment Conference statement.* Bethesda, MD: NIH (available from: Office of Medical Applications of Research, NIH, Federal Building, Room 618, Bethesda, MD 10892).

Stunkard, A. J. (1958). The management of obesity. *New York State Journal of Medicine, 58,* 79–87.

Stunkard, A. J. and Wadden, T. A. (Eds.). (1983). *Obesity: Theory and Therapy*, (2nd ed.). New York: Raven Press.

Wadden, T. A. and Vanitallie, T. B. (Eds.). (1992). *Treatment of the Seriously Obese Patient.* New York: Guilford Press.

CHAPTER 10: THE WELLSPRING PLAN FOR OVERWEIGHT CHILDREN AND TEENS: A PARENTS' GUIDE TO HEALTHIER, HAPPIER CHILDREN

Braet, C. & Van Winckel, M. (2000). Long-term follow-up of a cognitive behavioral treatment program for obese children. *Behavior Therapy, 31,* 55–74.

DeUgarte, D., & Slusser, W. (2010). Adolescent bariatric surgery in 2009. *Obesity and Weight Management, 6,* 39–42.

Gately, P. J., Cooke, C. B., Butterly, R. J., Mackreth, P., & Carroll, S. (2000). The effects of a children's summer camp programme on weight loss, with a 10-month follow-up. *International Journal of Obesity, 24,* 1445–1453.

Kelly, K. P., & Kirschenbaum, D. S. (2010).The promise of immersion treatment for obese children and adolescents in 2009: A review. *Obesity and Weight Management, 6,* 35–38.

Kelly, K. P., & Kirschenbaum, D. S. (2010, in press). Immersion treatment for childhood and adolescent obesity: The first review of a promising intervention. *Obesity Reviews.*

Kirschenbaum, D. S., DeUgarte, D., Frankel, F., Germann, J. N., McKnight, T. L., Nieman, P., Sandler, R. H., & Slusser, W. (2009). Seven steps to success: A handout for parents of overweight children and adolescents. *Obesity Management, 5,* 29–33.

Pratt, J. S. A., Lenders, C. M., Dionne, E. A. et al. (2009). Best practices updates for pediatric/adolescent weight loss surgery. *Obesity, 17,* 901–910.

ABOUT THE AUTHOR

DANIEL S. KIRSCHENBAUM, PH.D., ABPP, a clinical psychologist, was director of the Eating Disorders Program at Northwestern University Medical School, where he is professor of psychiatry & behavioral sciences. He is also the clinical director and vice president, clinical services, of Wellspring—a division of CRC Health (see wellspringweightloss.com)—and the director of the Center for Behavioral Medicine & Sport Psychology in Chicago. Dr. Kirschenbaum is a fellow and diplomate in Clinical Health Psychology of the American Psychological Association and former president of its Division of Exercise and Sport Psychology. He has served as a consultant to the United States Olympic Committee, the National Basketball Association, the Ladies Professional Golf Association, numerous professional journals, and several major corporations. Dr. Kirschenbaum has provided invited addresses at many professional conferences worldwide, received numerous grants for research, and published ten books and more than one hundred journal articles on weight loss, sport psychology, and related topics.